Take Back Time

Bringing Time Management to Medicine

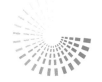

Judy Capko

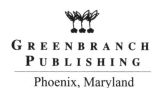

GREENBRANCH
PUBLISHING

Phoenix, Maryland

MATT
$54.95
8/09

Published by Greenbranch Publishing, LLC
PO Box 208
Phoenix, MD 21131
Phone: (800) 933-3711
Fax: (410) 329-1510
Email: info@greenbranch.com
Website: www.mpmnetwork.com, www.soundpractice.net

Printed in the United States of America by United Book Press, Inc. www.unitedbookpress.com

PUBLISHER
Nancy Collins

EDITORIAL ASSISTANT
Jennifer Weiss

BOOK DESIGNER
Laura Carter
Carter Publishing Studio

INDEX
Paul Hightower

COPYEDITOR
Kathleen McGuire Gilbert

Dedication

I dedicate this book to my husband, Joe—my greatest supporter.

TABLE OF CONTENTS

ACKNOWLEDGEMENTS

Thanks to my family and all the friends and colleagues that have encouraged me as I worked on this book. Most especially, I thank Vicki Dick, a dear friend who so generously gave of her time to read and critique the first draft, make editorial corrections, and provide accolades to keep me motivated. Of course, my thanks also go to the folks of Greenbranch Publishing, whose expertise contributed to turning the manuscript into a real book.

I pay tribute to healthcare professionals everywhere for their immense and tireless dedication and contribution to the field of medicine. I give my heartfelt thanks to each buyer of this book—I appreciate both your confidence and your support.

AUTHOR'S NOTE

To those clients and friends whose stories I have told, I have taken great caution to protect confidentiality and your identity without altering the important messages intended for the reader. Throughout the book the group size, specialty, career path, and name references are fictitious, but the stories are not.

For my readers, I promise you a very "real" journey in the hopes that you will grasp the opportunity to shed habits that destroy time so that you can find a path to higher productivity, a gain of personal time, and greater satisfaction at the end of each day.

Whether you are a clinician, executive, manager, or on the front line, a career in healthcare today requires you to face uninvited and constant change. Your days are filled with challenges and multiple stressors. I applaud each of you for your dedication to the field of medicine and other health services. Thank you!

Judy Capko

OTHER PUBLICATIONS BY JUDY CAPKO

Secrets of the Best-Run Practices

●

Secrets of the Best-Run Practices Audio Book

●

Toolbox Forms from *Secrets of the Best-Run Practices*

Available at www.mpmnetwork.com
or 800-933-3711

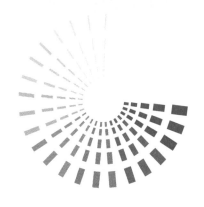

Introduction

*"You will never find time
for anything. If you want time,
you must make it."*

Charles Buxton

N early 15 years ago my husband and I were traveling in the back woods of Slovakia. At that time there were very few automobiles on the road. We came upon an old man walking along the roadside and offered him a ride. After driving about twenty miles, we spotted a policeman giving someone a ticket on the side of the road. Our rider, who seemed to speak no English, suddenly spoke up. He said, "Time is money." I was astounded that not only did he recognize the cost of someone getting a ticket for probable speeding, but was able to get the real message across quite eloquently using only three words. Yes, time is money, and when we rush, procrastinate or fail to use it wisely, it will cost us plenty. This humble man had it all figured out.

MY PERSPECTIVE

I have discovered that some people are plagued with time management issues and never seem to get ahead of the game. You may be one of them. Then again, you may be one of those fortunate few that have a good handle on time and seem to get more done with less. Even so, it is likely that you are affected by how someone else uses time. We depend on other people, and if they have trouble meeting deadlines or keeping up with their work, it ends up sabotaging us. Everyone struggles with time in one way or another, some more than others. The frustrations are very real.

This book is not a magic bullet, but it has lots of ideas for the medical professional to help keep the workforce more productive. It also touches on more personal issues concerning the importance of balancing your life and treasuring your own time. Perhaps this book will provide a little reinforcement, which is sure to be good for the soul.

When reading through the book you may identify with familiar scenarios and time situations you've already conquered. Just the same, no matter how well we seem to manage time, gentle reminders help us stay on track. Let *Take Back Time* serve as a refresher course—an opportunity to strengthen good time habits, find ways to deal with bad habits, and to become more disciplined with time. This is also a great "pass along" book if there is someone you know that has difficulty managing their time.

In my many years as a healthcare practice management consultant, I have focused on helping medical practices and healthcare systems become more efficient and people more excited about their jobs. This requires physicians and administrators to look at their work differently and be willing to listen to an objective outsider critiquing the way the job is done. This isn't easy, and it certainly isn't a popular position for the consultant. It's kind of like being called in to tell parents their baby is ugly.

Smart physicians and managers don't expect to have the perfect practice, but when they bring in a consultant they hope to obtain recommendations that, when implemented, will result in a well-run practice that is not wasteful of time or resources. How productive people are with their time has an incredible impact on efficiency, customer service, and overhead expenses. Guiding healthcare practices to become top performers, while honoring and appreciating everyone's contribution to the success of the business, is the consultant's mission.

The foundation of an efficient practice is the best allocation of time—reducing errors and eliminating waste, duplication, and unnecessary steps. It inevitably results in better cost management; improved service; happier patients, staff, and physicians; and though not perfect, a stellar practice.

Time is at the epicenter of our lives and in many ways dictates what level of success we will achieve, whether we're measuring personal satisfaction, professional accomplishments, or financial comfort.

TIME AND THE DOCTOR

The California Medical Association conducted a study of the top challenges of being a doctor today. Nearly half (46%) of the physicians said it was the long hours. Is it not enough time, the way time is spent, or both? Something has to give!

Just today I met with a young primary care physician who told me he is suffering from burnout. "There just aren't enough hours in the day," he said. "Everyone wants a piece of me and there's just not enough time to go around." Wow—this from a physician who has been in practice less than ten years. If he doesn't gain control over how he manages his day and time, how will he feel in another ten years?

When I probed further about how he spends his day, it became evident that his work patterns were classic for an inefficient medical practice. Paper processes and unnecessary steps are his norm, and the doctor is assuming responsibility for clerical and clinical tasks that don't require his expertise. He described a recurring problem with staff inconsistencies and errors resulting in too many processes, duplication, and reworks that contribute to his running late and rarely getting out of the office on time.

These inefficiencies cause him to spend time double-checking what has been done. He outwardly admitted his lack of confidence in staff and unwillingness to offload work to staff because of this. What a disaster! To top it off, there are five physicians in the practice and each one does things his own way—with his own staff. I know some of you can identify with both the frustration and the inefficiency this causes.

The practice was also way behind the curve with bringing in technology. In fact, the appointment scheduling system wasn't even automated. This troubled practice is losing out on opportunities to improve time management and to increase both efficiency and profits. They need to change the way they operate, get on track, and put time on their side.

THE TRUTH ABOUT TIME

Time is that elusive and priceless commodity of which there is never enough. You can't save it, buy it, borrow it, or replace it. We can, however, grasp it by making the most of our resources, eliminating unnecessary steps, and taking advantage of technology to streamline work processes and move information quickly.

Some experts give us something to think about when they tell us that it's not about managing time, it's about managing ourselves. Time is not the enemy. This may be true in theory, but let's face it, we all talk about time management as though time was an object, and in a way it is. It's that very object we can't seem to get our arms around.

ABOUT THIS BOOK

Take Back Time is a little book with a big purpose—to help you master time. It's not about cramming as much as you can into each day; it's about feeling good at the end of the day, knowing you made the best use of your time. It is an exploration of daily life in the healthcare arena, taking a look at the things that disrupt our time or make it nearly impossible to stay on time. My hope is that you will learn new ways to capture time and increase your own sense of fulfillment, both on and off the job.

By reading this book you will discover the key factors that can contribute to both abusing time and improving the way we manage it. The payoff for better time management is big: improved productivity, better financial results, and a calmer environment. To top it off, our lives become less stressful and there is a higher level of physician, staff, and patient satisfaction. It is bound to make for a better workplace and a better life.

Take Back Time will review how we use our time, what steals it away, and what we can do about it. Chapter 1 provides an introspective look at all those things that can sabotage your time. Communication is the focus of chapter 2, and the important role communication plays in better time management. Chapters 3 and 4 talk about two of the major contributors that make managing daily workloads and staying on time difficult: the telephone and the scheduling system. The cost of poor quality comes to the forefront in chapter 5, as you learn how to reduce variables to achieve better outcomes. Tips on developing a highly productive staff are reviewed in chapter 6, while chapter 7 discusses the use of technology to give people tools to get the job done better for less—less time and less expense.

You will find chapter 8 interesting; as it helps you understand the way patients think and demonstrates ways to "help patients help the practice." Chapter 9 provides insight on how to mine the business, using critical data to guide decisions and employ some smart planning techniques that help in preparing for the future. My favorite chapter is chapter 10, "Get Back Your Life!" It is intended to help ensure there is a healthy balance in your life, so you can reach your full potential and make the most of each day. The final chapter provides an understanding of what can be gained by making a commitment to change those habits that contribute to your feeling like there just *never* is enough time.

If some things seem repetitious between chapters, it's because they are. These are things that I believe are simply worth repeating, emphasizing, and reinforcing.

IN THE END

There are suggestions in this book that, if applied, can change your life. Sure, you've heard some of this before. Just the same, I can tell you from my years of experience working with professionals, a lot of you just aren't doing many of these things! It's just so easy to fall prey to old habits that kill your time. Perhaps *Take Back Time* can encourage you to reduce the time traps that are getting in your way so that there will be more time to do what you do well, fulfill your passions, and enjoy life more.

With the help of this book and your own ingenuity and determination, I trust that you will look at each day in a new way. Savor each day and end each feeling grateful for what has been achieved rather than feeling exhausted and frustrated by work that is left undone. Save the day—master time and reap the rewards.

IT'S UP TO YOU!

This book is small, but it is mighty. Take it seriously. Examine your own behavior and attitude as they relate to time. Challenge yourself to discover what you and the people you work with can do differently to master time.

You have the ability to capture time and make better use of it. It is likely to mean changing attitudes or habits, or perhaps changing structure and procedures, and learning new ways to work so that you can reduce the variables that disrupt tasks and take up more time. The effort is worth it, and no one can make it happen for you. It's up to you!

> *"The future is something which everyone reaches at the rate of sixty minutes an hour, whatever he does, whoever he is."*
> Clive Staples Lewis

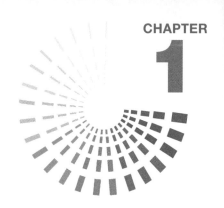

Are You Being Sabotaged?

"A habit cannot be thrown out the window. It has to be coaxed down the stairs one step at a time."

— *Mark Twain*

Imagine the perfect work day. Many of you do—on your way to work, you picture all the things you plan to accomplish during the day.

During a perfect day everything goes as planned and time is mastered, not wasted. Visualize it: you walk into the office and everything is calm and orderly, and everyone is in control and performing their jobs without confusion or disruption. You go to your office ready to start your day and work through it with ease, completing your goals. Mission accomplished! We are satisfied with a job well done! Sounds good, but it rarely happens. Usually it is just a forgotten dream. Too many days end with us feeling as though our time has been sabotaged. But has it?

Each one of those wild days begins with the best of intentions and an ambitious fantasy of what will be accomplished. So what gets in the way? When work is left unfinished at the end of the day or if we don't have time to pursue our goals, we become frustrated and discontented. This book's purpose is to help you identify the ways time can be compromised and to present solutions that work.

Perhaps unexpected circumstances continually emerge that need your attention, or certain people lean on you more than others. It could even be tangible aspects of the physical environment. After all, if we don't keep the building and equipment up to par we are sure to be caught in the crossfire when they fail to meet our needs.

Let's look at what can go wrong, the typical factors I've seen that sabotage time.

A LACK OF STRUCTURE

A solid infrastructure influences everyone's time and should be designed based on how the practice functions and what is expected of everyone. Too many practices run "by the seat of their pants." Everyone in the practice has a job, and for the most part, they pitch in to help each other. But this is often done without clearly defined responsibilities or boundaries of authority. Without structure it is difficult to determine the root cause of declining productivity (lost time), or to be prepared for unexpected shifts in work flow or volume. Without structure, time is not always used wisely.

The Organization

It starts with developing an organizational chart, often referred to as the "org chart." The org chart is a portrait of the practice's staff plan. It defines the primary functions of the practice and represents the line of authority and the responsibilities for each member of the office team: doctor, administrator, line managers, and clinical and clerical staff. The org chart will vary from practice to practice. The larger the practice, the more elaborate the chart, each intended to reflect the practice's operational structure and how decisions are made. In other words, who is the "go to" person for each position in the office?

It makes perfect sense for each practice to have an org chart; but frankly, in my more than twenty-five years of consulting, only about 15% of the practices I consult with had an org chart when I arrived on the scene. And for those that do have an org chart, a fair number of the charts seem to have been created in the dark ages and don't accurately portray the practice's structure. As a practice grows and positions are added or changed, it is important to revise the org chart to reflect those changes.

The People

Each person who works in the practice needs a clear understanding of what is expected of them on the job. At the same time, the physician and the manager need to be sure employees have the right skill sets for their jobs. This is accomplished through the careful and deliberate process of developing well-defined job descriptions (JDs) that clearly explain the primary tasks of each position, as well as the education, skill set, and amount of experience an applicant would need in order to be considered for the job. The JD becomes a powerful tool when recruiting for a position. It keeps you focused on the specific criteria for the job, thus removing emotion and subjective factors that can lead to selecting someone under- or overqualified for the position.

Once job descriptions are in place it's important to review and update them from time to time. Here are a few ways to keep JDs current and relevant.

- Each year on a particular date (say April 15th—easy enough to remember) give each person his job description. Ask staffers to review their own JDs and make notes to reflect any changes in what they do. To help staff succeed with this exercise, communicate its importance and provide each person with the following list of questions to address in relation to their position and responsibilities.
  - What technology has been added this past year that changes the way I perform my job?

○ Are there workflow or facility changes that impact what I do?

○ Have some of my prior responsibilities been shifted to another department or individual?

○ Are there tasks in my job description that have been eliminated?

○ Does my position now require additional training or education because of increased legislation, quality initiatives, or other practice needs?

Give them no more than five days to return the JDs or it will be a forgotten project, and you are likely to end up either hounding staff or becoming terribly frustrated.

• When an employee is planning to leave and has given you her notice, meet with her to review the JD and determine if changes are needed, or if a shift in responsibilities would improve the work flow or result in a better distribution of the workload among team members.

• When the practice grows, such as adding a remote secondary location or ancillary services, or bringing in a nurse practitioner, physician assistant, or another physician, make sure to update JDs. Take time out in advance to look at what additional staffing will be required, and look at the entire staff plan, including how the positions currently coexist and how they might change. Before creating a new position, examine the distribution of the workload to make sure you are creating an efficient position that meets the needs of the entire practice. This may mean removing tasks from several employees and shifting those tasks to the new employee. This might provide an opportunity for you to assign more challenging responsibilities to someone who excels and is worthy. Such a scenario is a perfect example of several peoples' jobs changing with growth. When this occurs, make sure JDs are reflected to show those changes.

COMPROMISED ENVIRONMENT

Take a good, hard look at your work environment: the facility, the furniture, and the equipment. The arrangement of work stations, the access to and placement of working tools such as computers and phones, and ergonomics are critical to being efficient and mastering time.

A few months ago I visited a busy gastroenterology practice and watched the staff at work. There were four people in the billing and reception area, and none of them were staying at their stations. They were playing musical chairs, rotating from station to station. I asked the manager why and was told that even though all four employees had their own computer, only one had Internet access. Give me a break!

You may be concerned that access to the Internet will result in staff spending time doing personal activities, or that the cost to get everyone online will be burdensome. In this situation, the price of lost productivity without Internet access is huge.

First of all, if employees are going to engage in personal activities they will do so without being online. It's your job to provide leadership and a work environment that keeps them motivated and productive. Secondly, the lost productivity for this constant game of musical chairs costs plenty. Think of the interruptions created by taking people off-task to wait for a shared terminal. Think of the unnecessary steps that are required. Think of the lost time for employees to refocus when they go back to their own work stations.

A time and motion study proved that this practice was losing thirty minutes of productivity for each hour because they were sharing an Internet-connected terminal. Based on an hourly pay rate of $20.00 with taxes and benefits, this cost the practice $20,000 a year. That's significant.

Another facility I visited had a well-organized structure. They hired a very capable and confident triage nurse. They gave her great clinical protocols approved by the physicians so she knew just what calls she could handle, with whom to schedule an appointment, and which patients to refer to the physicians for disposition. This was great. The problem was that the location of the medical records was a long distance from her triage station. A round trip from her station to retrieve a patient's record took ninety steps and required her to abandon the triage line, increasing the number of calls that were forwarded to her mailbox and had to be retrieved and returned. This was both time-consuming and inconvenient. The time to retrieve charts and return the calls that were waiting in her mailbox represented an estimated $8,000 annually in lost productivity. Of course this problem would be eliminated with an electronic medical record, referred to as EMR or EHR (to be discussed in chapter 7).

The Facility Audit

I suggest you audit the work environment for yourself and for the staff. Give it a critical eye and think about efficiency in terms of steps and time. Based on my past experiences, here are some typical time-wasters for you to consider as you conduct the environmental audit.

1. Too few copy machines. Copy machines are not that expensive, and when employees use one more than ten times a day, it should be within fifteen steps of their work station.

2. Printing encounter forms in the reception area when patients are checked in. It's a great idea to have the receptionist generate the charge ticket, but don't have it print at the reception station. Send it to a printer located at the nursing station. This provides a nonverbal signal of the patient's arrival for the nurse and keeps the receptionist from getting up from her station to retrieve and route encounter forms.

3. Physicians not having a work station at the hub of clinical activity: near the exam rooms and the nurse's station. When physicians are working out of their private office during the day, they may be moving too far away from where they actually treat the patients. As my friend Dick Haines, an architect with Medical Design International in Atlanta, Georgia, says, "Let the work come to the doctor." And he is right. It's important to minimize the steps clinical providers take while working; close proximity makes a big difference by the end of the day. Add up the steps taken by multiple providers and you'll see what I mean.

4. Not enough phones in the clinical setting. When a nurse and physician are jockeying to use the same phone, one of them is bound to wait.

5. No lighting signal system. This nonverbal communication system allows the physician to call for a nurse without leaving the exam room. It also lets the staff know which room the doctor is in. Some practice management software programs offer room monitors, but not all of these are easy to use, and many add more processes and end up being more time-consuming than a lighting system.

6. Non-standardized room set-up. Physicians and nurses work more efficiently when they do not need to leave the room for supplies and when the exam rooms are set up identically.

7. Not enough exam rooms. When physicians are unable to see a patient that has arrived at the office because there are not enough rooms, or several rooms are "shared" and not available, the physician will lose valuable time.

8. Too many exam rooms. Don't use exam rooms as a sub-wait station for patients. It's not fair to the patient and deludes you into thinking you are on schedule because fewer patients are in the reception area. During clinical hours one of the following activities should be happening in

every exam room: the nurse should be setting up the patient and taking his or her history, the patient should be dressing or undressing, the patient should be receiving clinical care, or staff should be preparing the room for the next patient. The number of exam rooms should depend on the physician or other healthcare provider's style, patient care issues, and the speed at which the clinical staff works. Exam rooms represent your production and as such they should be a core of activity that generates revenue.

9. No private office for the manager. This is one of the greatest compromises a practice makes. The manager needs privacy to handle financial matters, conduct business, meet and counsel individuals, hold meetings, and store important papers. Without exception, this job cannot be done correctly without adequate space.

Office Design

When designing a new facility it's worth the investment to hire an architectural firm that specializes in medical facility design. Select an architect who will conduct a pre-evaluation of your functional needs (or is willing to work with a consultant to accomplish this), assessing how the practice works, the flow, and how the facility can be efficiently designed to meet your needs and save everyone steps. Your space is important to higher productivity and improved profits.

The most efficient clinical space I've seen is based on the hub and spokes. The hub is a dual station where the nurse and physician work when they aren't with a patient during clinical hours. The spokes represent the exam room space with the diagnostic testing or procedure room space in close proximity. Here's an example, but remember that your space needs to be designed based on your needs (Figure 1).

PLAN AND ORGANIZE

Disorganization means dysfunction. We've already covered areas of organizational structure, but personal structure is essential to accomplish the things that require your time and talent. Most physicians and managers feel the burden of too many demands on their time, but by having a better grasp of each day in advance, we are more prepared to deal with the day's activities and make better use of time. The decisions we make throughout the day will be an indication of how much we truly value our own time.

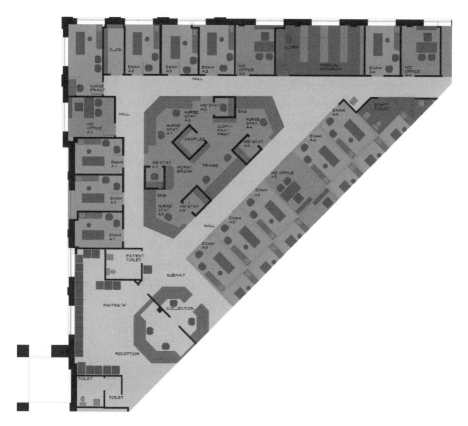

FIGURE 1. Sample Office Space Design
Source: Richard Haines, Medical Design International

The Pareto Rule

Busy administrators and physicians are faced with a broad range of responsibilities that demand their time, making it difficult to know which task to tackle first. Pareto's rule[1] says "80% of your troubles will come from 20% of your problems." The rule is named after Vilfredo Pareto, who in the late eighteenth century studied the distribution of wealth in Europe and found that 80% was held by 20% of the population. A number of published studies showed similar 80/20 relationships and claimed, for example, that "managers spend only 20% of the time to complete 80% of their work." These studies have resulted in Pareto's rule becoming an accepted part of management folklore.

---

[1] Juran, Joseph, *Juran's Quality Control Handbook*, New York City, NY: McGraw-Hill, 1988.

Pareto's rule suggests that situations you face rarely have equal impact or the same value and I agree. Some situations that are far less serious than others can end up consuming a great deal more energy and time. It takes focus and discipline to avoid such traps. You must weigh the value, decide which ones are the most important, and deal with them first. Rather than trying to deal with many trivial issues, select a vital few. The rule's value is that it reminds us to be selective in what we choose to do. In other words, evaluate the return on investment for the use of your time, which is a priceless commodity.

Project Management

Project management and time management go hand in hand. Applying project management principles improves your ability to manage time. It takes planning to a formal level by putting it in writing (Table 1).

Too often, we think we simply don't have the time to create written plans, but in reality this investment in time is worth it. There are many advantages to creating a written plan:

1. Saves time and helps you avoid obstacles that take up more time
2. Helps you to be realistic with the time needed to complete a project
3. Helps you identify the resources necessary to complete the project
4. Crystallizes your commitment
5. Defines expectations
6. Provides a guide to follow through completion of the project
7. Keeps you focused
8. Helps you to manage your time effectively

According to Dan Strakal, EdD, of Capable Consulting, the three key components of project management are (1) schedule, (2) budget, and (3) quality.

Once you have created a project plan, if any of the three components above changes, you can begin communication and negotiation. For example, let's say that you are expected to acquire an additional 2,500 square feet adjacent to your existing office space, and you have prepared a plan that allows you three months to accomplish this. If the physicians tell you they want to occupy this space in two months, something has to give.

In order to meet the new deadline you will be required to move up the target deadlines on specific tasks, which means that

1. you will need additional resources and the project budget will rise; or
2. you will not be able to equip or furnish the new space as originally planned, compromising quality.

TABLE 1. Sample Project Management Plan

Objective: Hire physician extender	Target Start Date	Target Completion	Assigned To	Costs
Clarify needs and costs • Determine scope of services • Develop job description • Research and develop salary schedule	February 15	March 1	Administrator, Medical Director	$0
Recruit • Create and place advertising • Conduct interviews • Conduct background checks	February 25	April 15	Administrator	$3,000
Select & Hire • Evaluate candidates • Prepare offer • Prepare contract • Offer hiring bonus • Prepare training schedule • Prepare clinical space	April 10	April 20	Administrator, Medical Director, Clinical Supervisor	$15,000
Planning & Orientation • Staff luncheon • Physician shadowing • Clinical supervision • Performance monitoring and evaluation	April 20	June 15	Medical Director, Clinical Supervisor	$6,000

You must communicate, negotiate, and agree on what is compromised and what the end result will be. It is unrealistic for the physicians or you to assume that any of the three components of the project will not be compromised when you make a major change or expectations shift.

Make Each Day Count

Start by planning each day. I'm a big proponent of the "To Do list." Some physicians and managers create a To Do list in their Palm Pilot or Blackberry. You can also store a list on your computer in Outlook Express or similar software that offers a daily schedule and task list. This makes it easy to refer to and you can even take a historical look at the past to assess how realistic you've been when planning your day. Some people still prefer a hardcopy list that sits on the top of their desk, and that's fine as long as it works for you. The important thing is making the list realistic. Even though many of you do this, I thought I'd share a few ideas on how to structure and manage the list.

A Time Plan

To make the most of each day, we must plan the next day's journey. This is best achieved by creating a Time Plan that orchestrates what you expect to accomplish. Begin your Time Plan by prioritizing activities so that the most important ones—those that have the greatest value—are at the top of the list.

Some activities may take only a few minutes, like scheduling that appointment with the lawyer to review a contract. Others may take hours, like preparing the financials for an executive committee meeting. For this reason, as you create the list, it's important to estimate the amount of time it will take to accomplish the task. Reserve 15–20% of your time each day for those unpredictable but necessary tasks that occur, and to regroup and plan for the next day.

Know thyself. I prefer to make quick phone calls first thing in the morning, because I'm more likely to reach someone and get it off my list. If the caller is not available, I'll ask him to return the call after 4:00 p.m. to ensure I tackle the rest of my list before I am interrupted.

If I think a call will be time-consuming, I'll make it at the end of the day when I've accomplished the other things on my list. I build my list based on the value of the activities and use time as a parameter for being realistic about what can be accomplished so that I don't get derailed. I group all the tasks that take less than ten minutes each and tackle them in the afternoon, once I have the high-priority time-consuming items finished.

Whenever you need to make a choice, apply Pareto's rule and your laundry list will be composed of items that are important, need your attention and will give you a sense of accomplishment.

Self-Inventory

Do a self-inventory to determine how well you manage your time. Over the period of a week to ten days take a look at how you plan your day, whether it's that To Do list or just a mental process of planning the next day's events. How many of those tasks are actually being accomplished, how many are being dismissed or forgotten, and how many are being bumped to the next day? Were you realistic in the amount of time allotted for the various tasks on the list?

If you are accomplishing less than 90% of what you set out to do, something is wrong. It could be overly ambitious plans—being unrealistic. It could be events, people, habits, or environmental issues that get in your way. Whatever it is, it's sabotaging your time. This book is intended to help you discover the problem and grasp a solution so you can make the most of each day.

Your Workspace

Now, check out the top of your desk and examine what is on it. How much of this is really necessary? Sure, it's all there for a reason, but does it make sense? Organize your desktop so that the things you use throughout the day are at arm's reach. Things that are not used on a daily basis should be removed from the desktop. A pending file and in/out boxes are excellent tools to keep you organized, but the only project on your desk should be the one you are working on. Be clutter free!

Now, how about the rest of the room? Are there stacks of magazines you plan to read, but just don't get around to it? If they've been there more than a few weeks they need to be discarded. When a periodical first lands on your desk, look at the table of contents. If there's something of interest, pull the article out and discard the magazine. Take one hour weekly to go through the stack you've created during the week. Read the first two paragraphs of each article; if it doesn't grab you, toss it. Create a reference library on your computer. Once you've read an article, if you think you'll refer to it later, scan it into the computer; otherwise, toss it.

How much paper is really necessary? If your own documents are in a well-organized filing system on the computer, why have hard copies of the same documents? When you need to retrieve a file you can just look at it on the computer. Only print it when you need to share the information with someone else by distributing a copy or reviewing the document in a meeting. You will always need some paper files, but it's amazing how much paper can be eliminated by storing things on the computer where they are easily accessible. It's just a matter of changing habits and becoming more organized.

LACK OF DISCIPLINE

Ouch! This sounds like a criticism, but it's not. I'm not talking about a lack of discipline in your life, I'm referring to time discipline—how you use time. I believe that even the most disciplined people sometimes fall into the trap of letting something or someone sabotage their time. I'm certainly no exception. I think the key is to recognize it when this happens and find out why. What culprit sabotaged your time? Once you find out, you can take action to keep history from repeating itself.

Interruptions

It's impossible to eliminate interruptions altogether, but there are ways to manage interruptions. Set criteria for acceptable interruptions so you aren't interrupted unnecessarily for something that can wait. Over the years when conducting efficiency studies, I have been amazed at how often I see physicians and administrators getting interrupted needlessly. Inevitably, it's just a habit, but sometimes it's a matter of micro-managing. Either way it kills time, and it's unhealthy for the practice.

Why do I say it's unhealthy? Because staff becomes too dependent on you, and they don't learn to resolve minor problems on their own. If we solve our employees' problems, they don't use their ingenuity and they lose confidence in their capabilities—not a good thing.

Ask yourself these key questions:

- Does staff interrupt me with something that can wait?
- Does staff come to me to get answers to problems that they could easily solve by themselves?
- Do I trust staff enough to let them make decisions that don't really require my input?
- Do I place boundaries on when staff may interrupt me?

An open door policy will steal your time. Set some ground rules to limit when it's okay for staff to interrupt you. For managers, I suggest establishing a window of time each morning and afternoon when you will allow interruptions, for example between 11:00 a.m. and noon and/or 4:00–4:30 p.m. Also define what types of interruptions are acceptable. Set some parameters that will reduce outside interruptions such as drop-in pharmaceutical reps and telephone calls that are non-emergent or not business-related. Let someone take a message and you return the call at your convenience!

If you establish ground rules and enforce them, staff will learn to value your time and understand what really needs your attention, what can wait, and what they can take care of on their own. You will encourage staff to be problem-solvers, and everyone benefits.

Value time more—eliminate unnecessary interruptions!

Procrastination

If you are a victim of your own procrastination it's costing you plenty. Procrastination results in a lack of planning and poor preparation. You end up reacting to circumstances and events and fall prey to crisis management. When this happens it compromises a quality result and we end up fixing what went wrong or duplicating efforts.

Honoring the To Do list helps reduce the tendency to procrastinate. Procrastination then results from bumping a task from your to do list and putting it off. Sometimes a bump is necessary. It can be caused by a domino effect when someone else's deadline prohibits you from accomplishing your objective. It can also be caused by a true emergency that takes priority. It's important to recognize the root of procrastination. It could be one or any of the following.

1. Ill-preparedness
2. A dreaded task
3. Uncertainty about how to approach a task; or objective is not clear
4. Not enough (or not the right) resources
5. No support from staff or leadership
6. Not committed
7. Low-priority task
8. Unrealistic expectations
9. Resisting change

Once the cause of procrastination is clear, something can be done about it. Perhaps it is best to forget it all together, which requires discussion and a decision with those affected by eliminating the action. The best solution may be to turn the job over to someone else or to calendar it for a later day. Perhaps it is one of those *trivial many* rather than those *vital few* that are worth your time. One thing is for sure: if a task keeps getting bumped, stop procrastinating and take action. Rid yourself of the procrastination habit and you will find new freedom to use your time in a way that makes sense.

Crisis Management

When I think of crisis management I can't help but think of one of my past clients. It was a busy neurosurgery group practice that was renowned for its diversity and innovation. The senior physician, whom I'll call Dr. Daily, was brilliant but also egocentric, and he micromanaged every aspect of the practice. The administrator was a very capable young man who simply wasn't given the authority to do his job and was constantly being undermined. The result was chaos and crisis management that took up everyone's time. The staff called it "a crisis a day" and they were just about dead-on. Nearly every day Dr. Daily would have something that he thought was critical, and he would bring down the whole staff in the middle of the day, calling everyone into a meeting. No one could get their work done. Productivity plummeted and overtime was excessive. Physicians didn't see their patients on time and were left with piles of work at the end of the day. This is certainly an extreme example, but crisis management results in poor use of resources, lower productivity, higher stress, and higher costs, with no or little improvement in the end result.

If emergencies in your practice seem to erupt frequently and result in crisis management, it's time to analyze those emergencies and their causes. If they aren't true emergencies they need to be put on the schedule and planned to prevent them from disrupting workflow.

My approach to solving this problem is to lay the facts on the table and get the stakeholders' attention.

1. Outline the financial costs. In this example, the cost for a two-hour meeting was allocated based on physician and staff wages and benefits. Here's a look at what it was costing this three-physician neurosurgery practice.
   - Per-hour cost for a total of eleven staff members (forty-hour week) = $209.00
   - Per-hour cost for a total of three physicians (sixty-hour week) = $553.00
   - Total costs per one-hour meeting: $762.00
2. Determine the emotional impact that may trigger even greater costs, such as high turnover. According to the Human Resource Management Society, it can cost as much at 150% of an annual salary to recruit and train a replacement for a position in your office. There is also the impact of lower staff morale and productivity. Conducting a staff satisfaction survey may provide supporting data regarding the trickle-down costs of these disruptions.

3. Find a champion among the stakeholders who will provide essential support to lead the cause.
4. Develop an intervention plan that offers several possible solutions and outlines the steps to get there.
5. Build in points of accountability that provide a punitive call for action.
6. Identify which members of the leadership team are best suited to deal with the offender.
7. Set a target date to meet with the offender and present your plan.

One physician or one administrator will not be able to resolve this without obtaining a consensus of support from the leadership team, but laying out the financial cost of crisis management is sure to get their attention. It may be politically smart to bring in an objective third party to intervene, such as your accountant or a skilled management consultant that has experience dealing with individuals who cause disruption. Most of the time the disruption is not intentional, but nonetheless, it will play havoc with the practice and everyone's time.

The Monkey on Your Back

Does someone else's work end up on your desk? If so, the monkey on his back becomes the monkey on your back. When the work you have planned for the day seems to grow with tasks that should belong to someone else, you've been sabotaged.

I've seen the warning signs. When someone tells me she's a "hands-on" manager it may mean she's doing work that doesn't require her attention or expertise. This sometimes happens when a manager has been elevated from the ranks. She was a receptionist, surgery scheduler, and biller. Because of this, she is expected to pitch in when others need help. In an urgent situation that's understandable, but too often it becomes a habit. The staff tends to lean on the manager for non-management tasks—and so do the physicians! When this happens a manager leaves important work unfinished so she can help out, which is a poor use of her resources.

This also occurs when a manager wants the staff to realize he's not an ivory tower manager, but someone that is willing to "pitch in." You may be willing, but it should only happen in an emergency. Make it a rare exception, not a pattern that keeps repeating itself.

I was recently in a six-physician OB-GYN office where the manager was sitting at the exit station processing a patient. She told me that the receptionist responsible for this was on her break and she was filling in. Unacceptable! The receptionist has breaks every day, so there needs to be a better plan that calls on another staffer to meet this need, not a manager! If you are a roll-up-the-sleeves manager, take a good, hard look to see if someone else's monkey is landing on your back. ●

TAKE BACK TIME

- *Create organizational structure and define staff responsibilities.*
- *Make your facility work to reduce steps and improve productivity.*
- *Keep staff at their desk with non-verbal communication.*
- *A self-inventory will help determine what steals your time.*
- *Do not let things and people sabotage your time.*
- *Remember the Pareto rule.*

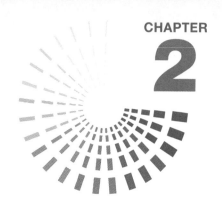
Can We Talk?

"The single biggest problem in communication is the illusion that it has taken place."

—*George Bernard Shaw*

Can we talk? These words may strike fear in your heart. Just think of the internal dialogue that it brings to your mind:

- There's a problem I don't want to hear about.
- I need to listen—this could be serious.
- Oh no, not again!
- Now what?
- This is bad.
- I don't have time for this.

Unfortunately, the question seldom brings enthusiasm or evokes a feeling of "I'm so glad you came, so I can hear what's on your mind." But communication isn't all about talking; it's about listening as well.

WHAT IS COMMUNICATION?

The definition of communication is "A giving or exchanging of information, signals or messages by talk, gestures or writing," according to the *New World Dictionary*. Everyone communicates. That doesn't mean we are good at it, and it doesn't mean the signals we give and receive are not misinterpreted. One thing is a fact: when communication is not clear or we deliberately avoid it, we are headed for trouble. This kind of trouble will be a sponge that absorbs a lot of time.

Effective communication gives us an excellent opportunity to use time wisely to motivate people, give directions, provide education, and make decisions that make a powerful difference in what we achieve.

Albert Mehrabian, PhD, is a professor that devoted years of study to communication. Dr. Mehrabian[1] declares communication to be 7% words, 38% tone of voice, and 55% body language. Thus we have the expression, "actions speak louder than words."

The Power of Gestures

Never underestimate the way you deliver a message—the gestures you use. If 55% of our communication is not what we say, but what we do, we need to be far more aware of our body language. Just think about different images and the impressions they create in your mind. For example, if you meet with someone and he sits down with his arms crossed, that's a huge message.

Mehrabian, PhD, Albert *Silent Messages*, Belmont, CA, Wadsworth Publishing, 1971.

Without a word being spoken, this person is telling you he is guarded and resistant. In fact, he may be even a little suspicious of what you are about to say. It's quite the opposite when someone sits down, leans in and nods his head up and down as you speak. He is definitely listening and is open to whatever you are discussing.

We have lots of traditional body messages we recognize at a glance, for example, the thumbs up, the peace sign, the wave, and some signs that are objectionable or offensive. I bring these up to prove a point. Body language and signals send a strong message and have an immediate impact.

Attitudes change instantly when non-verbal communication signals are sent. They can be positive or negative. Here are a few positive techniques you can apply to keep communication open and flowing.

Be on equal ground.

This means one person should not be looking down on the other. It creates an illusion of power for the one that is at a greater height. If you are standing and the other person is sitting, take a seat. This may seem like a minor issue, but it's not. It can be condescending or threatening to the person who is at a lower height.

Be a wise listener.

Here's where body language brings strength and affirmation. Lean in when you are listening to someone speak, and listen with all your senses. Nodding indicates you are an attentive listener and encourages the speaker to tell you more. Saying an occasional "uh, huh" is affirming and lets the speaker know you are attentive and care about what is being said.

Observe the other person.

Observe a person's body language and respond to it. If you meet with Jeremy and he seems nervous, acknowledge it, don't ignore it. This will result in far better communication and a better understanding for both of you. Saying something like "Jeremy you seem a little tense, please make yourself comfortable."

Make Your Words Count

Although Albert Mehrabian's study reveals that words only represent 7% of our communication, the tone of voice accounts for 38%. That's substantial, so choose your words carefully and be careful how you say things so that you are heard and interpreted the way you intend. If people aren't paying attention to what you say or if they take offense, it's your job to fix it. Use the opportunity to analyze what you said and how you spoke so that you can be a better communicator in the future. Here are a few tips to help you in your conversations with superiors, coworkers, and patients.

Repeat, repeat, and repeat.

Say the listener's name repeatedly. This immediately sends the message that the listener is important and that you really care. Notice the difference it makes when you are at a checkout counter and the employee serving you calls you by name. You immediately see her as an ally. It's almost like she becomes your friend. So when cranky Winston Grouch comes into the office next week, give it a try by saying, "Good morning Winston, how are you today?" If he gives the typical, "okay," you can continue on. "I see you've lost some weight, Winston. That's great. Now, we need to recheck your cholesterol levels before your next visit."

When someone is giving you a message, repeating what has been said goes a long way in clarifying both the message and the intent. "Terri, are you saying if we shift to ten-minute increments in our schedule, we can eliminate double-booking?" This will solicit confirmation or further explanation if it is needed.

Be sensitive.

This is where the rubber meets the road when it comes to the words you choose, especially when a discussion will be sensitive or has the potential to become confrontational. Keep the focus on the issue and not the person. Here's an example. Let's say an error was made on the surgery schedule that caused havoc in the office and created quite a stir. Your job is to fix the problem, not the person, and your words should reflect this. Instead of going to the schedulers and asking, "Who made this mistake?" have a huddle with the schedulers and simply ask, "How did this mistake occur and what can we do to prevent it from happening again?" See how this takes the focus off the people and makes it less personal? This verbiage sticks with the issues and keeps you directed on getting to the solution— your real purpose. It also gets the scheduling team working collectively to contribute to the right outcome.

Validate the speaker.

You can provide reassurance and validation by giving positive feedback. Tyler wants to know what you're thinking, so let him know by saying something like, "Hey, Tyler, I really like your ideas. This sounds like something we should explore further. Thanks a lot."

Good communication is powerful and important both to achieving the desired results and to making good use of your time.

THE ART OF COMMUNICATION

Effective and healthy communication is part skill, part art. But, when a message is delivered or interpreted poorly, it can kill time. Poor communicators are a part of our life, but if we understand the poor communicator, we can develop techniques to improve the exchange of information. We can help the poor communicator improve.

Take a look at the variable types of poor communicators I describe and you will recognize the challenges involved in working with these people. I will offer ways to improve the dialogue with poor communicators and challenge them to give a clearer message that makes better use of time—yours and theirs.

The Talker

Behold the talker! He is so busy talking that he doesn't take time to *listen*. He has much to say, but much of it is unnecessary. You all know him, because he makes poor use of his time and abuses yours! Here is a perfect example.

Mark comes into your office to tell you about a problem he has, but he gives you too much information (TMI), minutiae, and unrelated details. You try to listen, but when he gets derailed, so do you. The problem is when Mark finally has something relevant to communicate, he's already lost you and you aren't listening. You are no longer engaged. Sound familiar? Mark needs to get to the point!

Dealing with Mark isn't easy, but you can take charge of the situation and improve your communication encounters with him. When Mark asks, "Can we talk?" it's important for you to have a planned response that keeps you in control.

Give Mark a time limit. Let Mark know you want to engage in a discussion, but put time parameters on it. Let him know he has whatever time you have to give him, but in my experience what needs to be said can usually be said in the first five minutes. Then it's your decision on how much further you want to take it. Next, come up with your pat phrase like "Get to the point," "Give it to me in fifteen words or less," "TMI," or "In a nutshell, Mark." This confines Mark's endless words and makes him focus on the primary reason for the communication exchange: delivering a message. Limit the talker's abuse of time. Help him learn to communicate better and get back to work, thereby improving the use of his own time.

The Avoider

We think of the avoider as someone who is passive-resistant and even manipulative. Sometimes this is accurate, but there are those cases where people are not conniving; they simply have trouble dealing with conflict. Let's review a typical scenario.

Stacey has something on her mind, but instead of coming right out with it, she waltzes around the subject or adds a statement of justification. Stacey and Caitlin are both responsible for handling incoming telephone calls, but Caitlin is having some personal issues, spending a lot of time on personal calls and leaving the bulk of inbound calls for Stacey to handle. Stacey comes into your office and tells you she can't keep up with the phone calls. Then she goes on to tell you it's not Caitlin's fault, the phones have just become unmanageable. Herein lies the problem. Stacey wants to avoid the conflict of dealing with Caitlin's failure to support the incoming phone lines. Stacey doesn't want to solve the problem, she just wants you to make it magically disappear (without conflict) once she tells you about it. She's giving you limited information and expecting an easy fix, which is not realistic.

Your next step in dealing with the avoider is to probe for more. It's a matter of keeping an open mind and finding a way to gather more information. Probing can be accomplished by using the right words without pointing a finger. Saying, "Stacey, help me understand the situation," will get you where you need to go. Saying, "What are you trying to tell me, Stacey?" may cause her to put up a defensive wall and retreat. You can help Stacey recognize that talking about areas of disagreement doesn't have to result in conflict. Approach the problem as it is presented from Stacey's perspective. Then gather the facts without changing the focus, while giving Stacey grace and affirmation.

The Silent Type

Silence can be deadly. The silent type will not come to you when something isn't working, whether it's a relationship or a job assignment. Inevitably, it will backfire on him. And if it backfires on him, it backfires on you. Physicians and managers need to be mindful of the silent type. Watch for changes that result from his inability to communicate his problem. There may be a change in attitude or job performance. This could be expressed with silent resistance, lower self-esteem, deterioration in performance, or isolation and pulling away from the team. These are signs that something's brewing and needs to be addressed. If you want to resolve a problem before it has a major impact on the practice, you will have to take the first step by acknowledging what you have observed and how it is impacting the practice. He will need support, encouragement, and tools that teach him to speak up. This can only be accomplished if adequate trust has been built between the two of you. Communication with the silent type will require careful planning and determination on your part, but the silence must be broken.

The Know-It-All

This person has the solution to everybody else's problems but never looks in the mirror to see what she is doing wrong. She always knows best and thinks everyone wants to hear what she has to say. Even when she has good ideas, nobody is listening. Regardless of the forum of communication, she needs to understand the power of minimizing her words and valuing the opinions and ideas of others.

The know-it-all has to be told to do more listening and less talking. She needs to understand that unsolicited opinions should be limited and take an example from her less vocal peers. Change her habit of constantly giving her opinion by stopping her at the pass. This is a time when interruption makes sense. "Jane, we've heard your opinion, now let's hear from someone else." You also need to meet alone with Jane and suggest that she bring her opinion to you before discussing it with everyone else. This will help guide her to change her approach to communication and learn to respect the opinions and time of the rest of the staff.

COMMUNICATE YOUR WAY

Keeping communication healthy and open is one thing, but we must also determine the best forum to communicate various types of information, whether it is sensitive, generic, or positive. The goal is timely, thoughtful, and healthy communication that makes the best use of our time.

The way you choose to communicate in different situations will be a reflection of what you value. Success depends upon your making the right choice in how to communicate. Read on.

Power Huddles

It works in football and it works for the practice—taking time to huddle. A huddle is an informal gathering to examine a situation, discuss strategies, and make decisions. There are a variety of opportunities to have a timely and effective power huddle.

The morning huddle is a great example. It's an excellent way for a team of people to communicate and start the day. The idea is to review the day's schedule and plan ahead. It provides an opportunity to explore potential problems or conflicts and identify actions that will minimize or eliminate those issues.

Here are a few examples. If David Evans was double-booked with a ten-minute appointment, but is a senior citizen with multiple problems, it's sure to cause delays unless the appointment is strategically rescheduled within the day. If an important lab report isn't in a patient's record, you can retrieve it before she arrives. If a new patient has insurance you don't accept, someone needs to call him in advance to let him know what his financial responsibility will be. Dealing with these issues in advance will save a ton of time, reduce commotion in the office, keep the doctor on schedule, and keep the practice humming.

Morning huddles are a great investment of time and a communication tool that works. It requires a commitment and it means getting into the office in time to have the huddle without compromising the schedule and getting off to a late start. The huddle typically takes less than five minutes.

Power huddles work in a variety of situations, such as a small team of people who want to develop a consensus before they begin a project, or refresh key points and recommendations before presenting a report.

Memos and Newsletters

A written memo does not replace other forms of communication, but there are times when it is the best way to communicate. Memos should be used as a bulletin to send out the same information to different people all at once.

A memo should be carefully crafted to ensure it communicates clearly and will not be misinterpreted. Such messages as a change in a staff meeting to another date and location, a change in a staff person's voice mailbox number, or an update on the call schedule work well with a written memo.

On the other hand, a memo should not be used as the initial way to communicate sensitive information, complicated instructions, or information that requires reinforcement of the message and its intent. A memo used for any of these purposes will add confusion and may be seen as an effort to avoid more personal communication. It may wind up becoming a disaster in which people end up standing around discussing the message, their view of it, and various interpretations. Be cautious as to how you use memos, and do not use them to replace communicating in person to individuals or to a group of people.

Electronic Messages

We are living in the age of technology and it certainly has changed the way we communicate. In fact, an entire chapter in this book will be dedicated to the use of technology in managing time. Electronic communication is a marvel that saves an unbelievable amount of time and helps you communicate in the office in real time. Intra-office e-mail and instant messaging are perfect ways to transmit information in real time with minimal steps. Electronic communication also provides a tracking tool for historical review or retrieval.

If the receptionist has a patient who is getting a little perturbed because of a longer-than-usual wait, she can instantly send a message to the nurse to find out what is causing the delay and how much longer the patient will need to wait. She can then communicate to the patient to relieve his anxiety, and the nurse will be prepared to apologize to the patient, comfort him further, and let the physician know what to expect. The biller can send a message to the receptionist when she spots a slow-paying patient on the schedule and either ask the receptionist to collect payment or have the patient wait to meet with a member of the billing staff before leaving the office. All this is done while staffers sit at their desks, saving time and steps while improving communication.

One-on-One

Anything that is confidential or sensitive to particular individuals, whether positive or negative, should be handled during a one-on-one conversation.

If it's not informal in nature, schedule it, plan for it, and do not allow interruptions. If you fail to do this you will not get the full advantage of the interaction. In fact, you will be discounting the value of the communication, implying that it is not important and may even sabotage the end result.

It's not important to have frequent one-on-one exchanges. What is important is having them when they are needed.

One-on-one meetings can be powerful, giving you the chance to learn more about an individual, to have him learn more about you, and to share viewpoints and both personal and practice objectives. Such communication can be the glue that keeps staff members wanting to work for you and taking ownership of their contributions with pride.

Meaningful Employee Meetings

Here are the most important things to remember about meetings with staff, whether it's the entire staff, one or two departments, or a committee. If you apply these five rules, you will have stimulating meetings that unite people and keep them motivated.

1. Have a defined purpose and goal for the meeting.
2. Be committed.
3. Have structure and stick with it.
4. Encourage full participation.
5. Manage the meeting.

Have a purpose.

Too often I hear staff complain that either they don't have regular staff meetings or that the meetings are worthless due to a lack of open exchange of communication, and nothing is really accomplished. This happens when the meeting does not have a defined purpose and is simply a routine obligation or habit that appears meaningless to the attendees.

If the supposed purpose of the meeting is for the manager or the doctor to give a report and tell staff what you want them to hear, there is no "real" purpose or need. It would be better to give this information in a written report. In fact, a staff meeting with one-way communication can be destructive. It can demoralize staff, making them feel like their input isn't important and their opinions don't count. They can become frustrated and angry. It splinters the ability to create or nurture group unity.

The meeting may have a specific topic as its focal point, such as discussing an upcoming computer conversion or planning for a new physician that is coming on board in a couple of months. Just the same, every meeting should have one common purpose: an exchange of information, open dialogue, and sharing opinions and ideas for the betterment of the practice. This central theme makes individual staff members feel that they are recognized for their contributions—that they are important to the practice. It helps keep the team unified and energized.

Don't have a meeting just because you meet the first Monday of each month. If there is no reason for the meeting and things are going smoothly, it may be better just to have a staff appreciation luncheon this time around.

Make a commitment.

Take time to properly plan for a meeting, give everyone advance notice, and get it on the books early.

Start and end meetings on time. Require everyone to be there when the meeting starts. Stop other office activity and do not allow visitors or non-emergency telephone calls to interrupt a meeting. Finally, don't cancel and reschedule meetings, except on rare occasions. It will send everyone a message that the meeting is not a priority, and neither are the needs of the people who were scheduled to attend.

Being committed also means involving the stakeholders. When it comes to staff meetings, at least one of the physicians should attend. In a group practice this can be done in rotation, so that each physician gets involved during the year. When it comes to a committee meeting that affects multiple departments, representation from each of those departments should be included. If it's an individual department meeting, everyone in that department should be there. They need to know what's going on and be involved; they need to listen, and they need to be heard.

Structure it.

Structure begins by defining the purpose of the meeting and developing an agenda that addresses that purpose. Take some time, plan the content of the meeting, and determine whether you want to invite someone else to give a report. This can be a great opportunity to share information. For example, if Michelle attended a seminar on billing regulations, it would be nice to have her share what she learned, informing everyone of regulatory changes that affect the practice and engaging in a discussion about how these changes can be implemented.

Prepare a written agenda three to five days in advance, and circulate it to the expected attendees. Invite them to offer suggested topics to include on the agenda. Of course, it will be your job to determine whether the topic is relevant and how much time should be dedicated to each subject of discussion.

A meeting action list needs to be developed (see Table 1). You can do this yourself or assign someone to be the meeting's recorder. List each action item, identify who is responsible for completing the assignment, and record the expected date for completion. At each meeting, the action list from the prior meeting should be reviewed and updated. This monitors activities and holds each person accountable for the tasks that have been assigned to him or her. Just as importantly, it keeps everyone informed and committed.

Manage it.

This is where talent and finesse come into play. You don't want to control the meeting, you want to manage it and lead the discussion. Follow the agenda, allowing a set amount of time for each agenda item. Make sure it is an informational exchange and not one or two people taking charge and monopolizing the discussion. Here are a few tips to manage meetings and make them more meaningful.

- Invite relevant staff members to give a report. For example, if collections have declined across the front desk, the billing manager can run a weekly

TABLE 1. Meeting Action List				
Type of Meeting _____ Date_____				
Description/Action Item	Person Assigned	Target Date	Actual Date	Comments

report comparing the dollar amount and the percentage of patients that have paid at the time of service for the past six weeks; he or she can also graph it to show the high and low points. This will surely result in discussion with the receptionists and perhaps some suggestions for improvement.

- Ask for feedback once a report or an opinion is given. Ask other people if they agree or have anything to add.
- Seek individuals out. When you observe certain staff members staying silently on the sideline or engaging in sidebar conversations, draw them out by asking, "Mary, do you agree with Martin?" or "Alicia is there anything you want to add to that?" or "Robert, how do you think this can be solved?"
- Follow the agenda. Refer to it to bring the focus back if the information exchange gets off on another subject.
- Review the action list. At the beginning of the meeting, review past assignments. At the end of the meeting, confirm new assignments.
- Thank everyone for their participation.

MAKE THE MOST OF IT

We communicate in many ways, and communication influences how we manage time and what we, as an organization and as individuals, accomplish. Communication is powerful and it's our job to make the most of it. ●

TAKE BACK TIME

- *Remember that body language and tone of voice account for more than 90% of what we communicate.*
- *Be a better listener to improve communication.*
- *Take steps to identify and help poor communicators improve their skills.*
- *Select the right forum for communicating to get the best result.*
- *You can have powerful meetings by following five simple rules.*
- *Healthy communication saves time.*

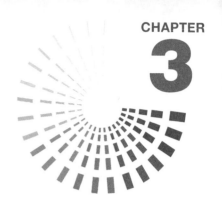

Telephone Madness

*"This 'telephone' has too many
shortcomings to be seriously considered
as a means of communication."*

—*Western Union internal memo, 1876*

What is telephone madness? It refers to those days when the demand on the telephones seems to rule the practice and destroy any hope of calmness. Chaos wins and everything else seems to go by the wayside. Yes, it is madness. It takes some effort to overcome the seemingly uncontrollable phones, but there are solutions that will open up time staff can dedicate to important tasks that get neglected when the practice is plagued by out-of-control telephone traffic.

Addressing how well a practice manages telephone demand is one of the more important factors in assessing how time is managed for the entire practice: the physicians, managers, staff, and even the patients. This is certainly reason enough to give telephone madness the attention required to resolve it.

FACE THE CHALLENGE

When the telephone demand exceeds the practice's capacity to handle it, disaster looms. The phone lines are tied up, the staff is inundated, work flow is impeded, and frustration mounts. Yikes! This is nothing new; it has plagued medical practices across the country for years, but it becomes more complicated with patients who are part of the "Now Generation"—people for whom cell phones are a life necessity and impatience rules the day. This attitude has expanded to become cross-generational, as society has access to more advanced technology, information, and instant communication. The consumer's expectations have become more demanding and they have high expectations. They are easily frustrated when these expectations are not met.

The Commitment

I recall an incident that took place at a physician conference last year when I did a presentation on managing telephone demand. Several physicians belonging to the same medical group approached me after the talk. They told me they had a serious problem with their phones. I asked them how they determined this, and one of the physicians said, "When I called into the office last week I was on hold for over ten minutes and it wasn't the first time!" That certainly is telling.

I probed further and discovered that this was a problem that had been going on for quite a while, and they were paying a very big price.

Patients were revolting, the physicians were upset, and staff was throwing up their hands in despair. Everyone was complaining, but no one was taking action. These doctors didn't know where to begin to fix the problem, so it was ignored and continued to grow. No one was willing to take responsibility and commit to facing the challenge head-on. Where there is no commitment, there is no solution!

Since a problem with telephone demand affects the entire practice, it is management's responsibility to involve everyone. The physicians and the manager must be willing to develop a plan and see it through from beginning to end! This takes time and resources in the beginning and it means monitoring compliance and accountability later.

LOOK AT THE DEMAND

Most practices struggle with peak times, when the volume of callers is very large. Peak times often cause major disruptions in both workflow and patient service. Examine past telephone demand for inbound calls to identify important peak volume patterns. Then measure it against your staffing capacity to handle this volume. This will help you to understand the depth of the problem. Here is an example.

I was recently in an office where telephone demand became a major problem. Two receptionists were assigned to check in patients and manage inbound telephone traffic. These two receptionists were checking in an average of 102 patients a day. Twenty percent of these were new patients. Add to this approximately 310 inbound phone calls a day and you get the picture.

It's impossible for two receptionists to manage that type of volume and not keep patients waiting—either on the phone or in the office. The check-in delays trickled back to the clinic, causing the physicians to fall behind schedule. This nightmare had a high price tag.

Let's look at the story these numbers tell.

Check in:

20 new patients × 4 min. each	= 80 min.
82 established patients × 1.5 min. each	= 123 min.

Inbound calls:

310 × 3 min. each	= *930 min.*
Total time spent on phone:	= 1,133 min.
	= 18.7 hours
	= 2.3 FTE* staff

Full time equivalent

No question about it, in this case demand exceeds capacity. Assume that these employees are engaged in other activities at least 10% of the time, and you can quickly see the problem. There are several different approaches that can be considered to meet this type of demand.

- Add more staff.
- Implement better systems.
- Reduce the number of inbound and outbound calls.

None of these approaches should be implemented without carefully studying the symptoms, diagnosing the problem, and selecting a long-term remedy, rather than a band-aid solution. Implementing better systems and reducing the number of calls are the most cost-effective strategies.

The Virtual Patient

The virtual patient is not on the daily schedule, but nonetheless demands and *deserves* your attention. Most of these patients call the office for a variety of reasons or special requests that staff must deal with during the day. If the practice is not equipped to deal with the typical volume of virtual patients, the demand increases. The virtual patients that are anxiously waiting for a call back from the practice will become restless and are likely to call in again. These repeat calls take up a lot of time and could be avoided if the practice was more responsive.

It becomes a Catch 22. The practice doesn't have time to respond because of the volume, yet the volume increases because they fail to respond to the initial calls. Then the practice is bogged down with repeat calls or with callers who were kept on hold, hung up in frustration, and called back. To stop this cycle, you must understand the types of call you are getting and find a better way to meet those callers' needs. There are some typical types of calls practices get from the virtual patient, and you have the ability to reduce these:

- Request a prescription
- Need medical advice
- Request test results
- Schedule an appointment
- Need referral or billing assistance
- Repeat calls

Track telephone activity for your practice for a period of several weeks to determine the type and volume of calls you receive. Table 1 offers a sample form, but you'll want to customize the study based on the typical reasons patients call your office.

TABLE 1. Telephone Activity Tracking Form

Time Frame	Appts.	Ins. Billing	Referral	Test Results	Hospital or MD	Rx	Other	Repeat Calls
7:00–8:00 a.m.								
8:00–9:00 a.m.								
9:00–10:00 a.m.								
10:00–11:00 a.m.								
11:00 a.m.– noon								
noon–1:00 p.m.								
1:00–2:00 p.m.								
2:00–3:00 p.m.								
3:00–4:00 p.m.								
4:00–5:00 p.m.								
5:00–6:00 p.m.								
6:00–7:00 p.m.								
TOTAL # OF CALLS								

Once you've gathered the numbers, graph them based on time parameters so you can visually analyze the peak demand and clarify the most frequent types of calls coming into the office. Take note if you are experiencing substantial repeat calls—either you don't have enough staff to manage the demand, or internal inefficiencies are causing a delay in responding to the initial call. These inefficiencies may result from poor training, poor compliance, or a general lack of accountability.

Figure 1 displays the distribution of phone calls throughout the day for a busy obstetrician/gynecology practice. The graph shows a burst of activity following the lunch break, an indication of pent-up demand created during the absence of lunch hour telephone coverage. There is also a spike in repeat phone calls between 3:00 and 5:00 p.m., which implies that calls made earlier in the day remained unanswered, resulting in repeat calls.

A Systems Problem

Evaluate your telephone system and its functions from time to time. Look at the capacity. Do you have enough telephone handsets, phone lines, and staff

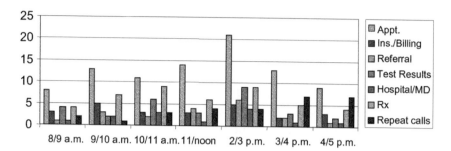

FIGURE 1. Telephone Traffic

to meet existing and future demand? Begin with a little investigative work to determine the features and capacity of the existing telephone system and whether it is expandable. You might be surprised.

It's quite common for staff to underutilize the capabilities of the telephone system. This happens when the people originally trained on the system are no long working in the practice. The people that follow usually learn only the rudimentary functions required to do their job at the time and think that's all the system can do. If you have auto-tender capabilities (that familiar automated voice that directs inbound phone callers) and aren't using them, you may want to start. For years physicians have resisted, considering the automated message and menus too impersonal for their patients, and they feared the patients would complain. Things have changed. Most businesses have applied sophisticated auto-tender telephone messaging for inbound calls, so the consumer has learned to accept this and adapt. Patients are no exception. If you are concerned about converting to an automated system, survey your patients. You just might be surprised at the results.

Another system problem can be an insufficient number of incoming phone lines to meet the demand. If patients are having difficulty getting through to you, you will need to identify the depth of the problem.

Find out if you can run reports on your existing system to determine the following:

1. How many calls are being abandoned—people that were kept on hold and finally hung up
2. Busy signals—people that couldn't get through
3. Peak volumes—times of day when telephone traffic is the highest

If your telephone system is not sophisticated enough to give you this information, check with your phone company's marketing department to see if they can conduct a lost-call and peak demand study. If not, you will need to resort to keeping a manual tab on inbound calls.

THE SOLUTION

Take heart, there's a solution to every problem. And in the case of telephone madness it's really a matter of analyzing your system's capabilities, your telephone traffic, and other contributing factors. This will enable you to identify the most appropriate solutions. The goal is to manage telephone demand without sacrificing patient service. This will result in reduced stress in the office and improved production—a magical combination!

Reduce Demand

Think strategically and you will be able to eliminate some calls altogether, reducing the burden on the system and the staff. Begin by tackling the demand and reducing the volume of calls. Then you will be able to clearly determine what system changes are required, such as the number of inbound lines, private lines, voice mail, direct lines, and menu options.

The Visit

When patients are seen in the office, handle whatever you can at the visit. For example, check their prescriptions and give them appropriate refills. If you have a diagnostic or consultation report, communicate the findings. Make sure the patient clearly understands the treatment plan and instructions. This will eliminate many patient calls down the road.

Here are a couple of slam dunks that will further reduce calls.

- Schedule follow-up appointments while the patient is in the office. This includes continued care patient visits, and post-op visits when the patient is having the pre-op exam. In pediatric practices, if you are seeing a pre-kindergartner in the spring, schedule the child's school physical for a few months later.
- When a patient is referred to a second physician, be sure to give patients copies of medical reports the other practice will need.
- Get patients' e-mail addresses for future reference and communication.
- Ask patients if e-mail is an acceptable way for you to communicate with them.

Before the patient leaves, probe to be sure you address their concerns and answer questions that may not have been asked. The physician, nurse, and receptionist should end each encounter by asking "Is there anything else we can do for you today?" Sure, this takes time, but it takes less time than getting a call later on that requires documenting the nature of the call, pulling the chart, returning the call, and filing the chart. Even in an electronic world, dealing with questions after an office visit takes more time. The more you manage at the time of the visit, the better!

The Internet

Get off the phone and onto the Internet. Make sure staff members who use the phone more than 20% of the time each day have their own computer terminals and access to "the Net." It's a far better way to communicate with referring practices, verify insurance benefits, and check on claims status. In addition, e-mailing is quickly becoming a preferred method of communication with technology-savvy patients. Using the Net saves time and reduces telephone traffic.

Staff can reduce phone use and stay at their desks by communicating with each other online through instant messaging and interoffice e-mail. This saves a lot of interruption and disruption in the office. It reduces processes, eliminates steps and saves more time.

Automation

If you are handling one-way communication with patients manually, explore ways to reduce those calls through an automated system. One-way communication systems are far more sophisticated than in the past and reduce the burden on the existing phone system. Here are some features that are now available for a fraction of the cost of managing these tasks on your own.

- Confirming new patient and routine appointments.
- Reminding patients to schedule return appointments, annual pap smears, mammograms, flu shots, repeat studies, and more.
- Providing scheduled patients with pre-appointment or pre-study instructions.
- Notifying patients of emergency cancellations.

It saves time and money to handle these tasks remotely, so start looking for a vendor with remote services that will best meet your existing and potential needs without using your phone lines.

The System

The analysis of inbound telephone traffic and system demands will guide you in developing the most appropriate solutions to telephone madness. Once you have reduced the actual demand, verify that you have enough incoming telephone lines to handle the volume. Then implement tools that support demand, reduce the burden on staff, and improve service. Most practices have a flexible telephone system with many features, including hands-free, intercom, speaker phone, headsets, the auto-tender, and the ability to track on-hold time (sometime referred to as "being in orbit").

Telephone Tree

When you first implement an auto-tender system, you will need to decide how to set up the most effective telephone tree. A good telephone tree will clearly direct patients in case of an emergency and makes it easy for callers to understand how to reach the person or department that can best serve them.

The menu options—branches on the telephone tree—should match the areas of greatest demand. Base this on the results of your telephone tracking study; it will save you from having callers bounced around, upsetting the patients and using up needless staff time to get the patient to the right place.

The menu of options should be limited to five. When there are too many choices, patients get confused and aren't sure which one to choose.

Voice Mail

Voice mail is an important adjunct to handling telephone traffic, but to succeed it must be well managed. This requires establishing firm response time guidelines. Work with the staff to determine parameters for responding to their voice mail, based on the nature of the calls. For example, you may decide that nurses should check their voice mail every half-hour, but you are comfortable with the billing department responding to calls within two hours.

Make sure the individual outgoing message on each mailbox lets the caller know when he can expect a response. For example, "This is Sally, Dr. Capko's nurse. I check my messages frequently and will respond to you within an hour of your call." Then it's your job to spot check mailboxes occasionally to analyze volume and ensure staff is compliant. Problems will be exacerbated if you don't hold staff accountable for responding to their voice mail without delay.

Message On Hold

It's impossible to eliminate having callers placed on hold, but when they are in the queue you can make them a lot more comfortable by occupying their time and educating them at the same time. Message on hold systems are perfect for this purpose. You can provide seasonal information, such as telling seniors it's time to get their flu shots, or during the summer reminding everyone to use their sunscreen and reapply it during the day. You can also offer timely medical alerts if confusing information has hit the media, if you simply want to give your patients facts about nutrition and exercise, or if you want to remind patients that your office has relocated. You will be giving better service that actually saves time. Just the same, this is not an excuse to ignore patients on hold. Thirty seconds is a long time, and one minute seems like an eternity when you are waiting on the telephone.

The People

Realistically, a receptionist cannot give both the arriving patient and telephone callers the attention they deserve, so move the phone traffic off the front desk to a quiet, professional, and private location. This can be in the business or clinical setting—whatever works logistically for you and does not compromise efficiency. For many practices this means change—looking at how the workload is currently distributed and modifying job assignments.

In a solo practice where the receptionist is the scheduler, it's not possible to move telephone traffic to another location in the office. In this case, make sure you have back-up for the receptionist when she is serving a patient or tied up on a phone call. The receptionist should not wear a telephone headset. It is insensitive to arriving patients and frustrates them.

Telephone Protocol

Develop telephone management protocols and train staff accordingly. For example, require every person who answers the phone to identify the practice and to give her own name. Staff should learn to repeat the patient's name during the conversation, obtain and maintain a rapport, and make the caller feel important. Develop staff telephone scripts to create continuity in what is being said. Scripts also help build staff confidence with handling telephone calls.

When it comes to responding to clinical calls, staff should know exactly what information to obtain on the intake, for example, not only what symptoms the patient has but how long she has had the symptoms and what other conditions exist. If the patient has a rash, is it red, does it itch, is it oozing, and does she have a fever? Physicians and nurses need to develop these protocols and train staff. It will reduce the number of calls required to gather information essential to assessing and treating the patient and will result in a quicker response. Be sure your telephone protocol prohibits staff from giving medical advice that has not been authorized by the physician.

Lunch Hour Debacle

Too many medical practices still shut down the telephones during the lunch hour. This is a big mistake. It results in far greater telephone traffic when the lines open up again and demand then exceeds capacity, making it near-impossible to stay on top of the workload.

Closing down your lines at lunch is also poor service. Many patients want to make their appointments on their own lunch break. If they can't reach your office, they just might go elsewhere.

Other service industries would never dream of closing down their phones at lunch. Why? Because being available opens the door to serve their customers better and to gain new business. Just think about it. Here's a scenario on the financial gains you might experience if two new patients were captured each week because of better phone coverage.

Assumption:

New patient net value $350 × 2 per week × 52 weeks = $36,400.00

Operate your practice like a business and keep the phone lines open. Not only is there potential to gain additional revenue, the existing patients will be happier, and staff will not be faced with the typical pent-up demand that occurs when phones are turned back on.

Billing Calls

Billing calls from patients can be a good thing—it generally means they want to pay you. Make it easy for the patient and the practice by having a direct phone number for the billing department, which should appear on the patient's statement. Also, cycle bill your patients, sending statements by alphabetical segments each week so that calls about the statements will be distributed throughout the month.

Take a critical look at the patient statement you mail out to be sure it is user friendly. It should be easy for the patient to understand how much of the balance is pending payment from the insurance company and how much the patient actually owes.

You can also use the billing statement to give patient information that can be keyed into the computer so that it prints on their next statement. For example, you can let patients know you have a new doctor on board or that you've opened a satellite office across town. Remember, any time you automate communication, processes are eliminated and time is saved.

THE LAST WORD

The patients have the last word, and if you don't meet their needs they will complain, or worse yet they will talk with their feet and move on to a competitor. When it comes to patients' primary complaints about telephone service, this is what they have to say:

- Put on hold too long
- Doctor was slow to call back
- Staff was discourteous
- Doctor never got back to me

I've given you some suggestions to alleviate these complaints. Now it's your turn—take action. Make sure the staff is properly trained on the telephone, give them the tools to do the job, and hold them accountable to performance criteria that support efficiency and consistency. Eliminate telephone madness and give patients the time they deserve. ●

TAKE BACK TIME

- *Get the facts: Examine types of calls and volume of calls.*
- *Reduce repeat calls through quicker response and better communication.*
- *Probe more at the patient visit to reduce calls later on.*
- *Develop a "sensible" telephone tree.*
- *Use automation for one-way communication.*
- *Get off the phone and onto the Internet.*
- *Set telephone protocols and hold staff accountable.*

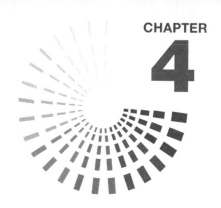

The Sensible Schedule

*"There cannot be a crisis today.
My schedule is already full."*

— *Henry Kissinger*

When it comes to challenges that eat away at our time and threaten patient satisfaction, the appointment schedule ranks near the top. In fact, its only competition for creating dissatisfaction and havoc in the medical office comes from the phones. Scheduling concerns can seem impossible to conquer. In fact, I have never heard a physician or manager tell me they have the answer for a perfect schedule. Perhaps the perfect schedule does not exist; nonetheless, every practice has the ability to create a sensible schedule.

It requires an investment of time to take a historical look at the schedule—finding out what is not working, understanding the implications (in both time and money,) exploring how scheduling can be more realistic, and making a commitment to shifting not only the way you schedule, but the way you *think* about the schedule.

START AT THE BEGINNING

First recognize the problem needs attention and quit putting your finger in the dike. Step back and take a new look at what is and isn't working—and why.

Look at the Indicators

Physicians, staff and patients all feel the results of an unmanaged appointment schedule. There's a sense of frustration, stress mounts, patients become more insistent and sometimes indignant. Everyone in the practice begins to feel they are working harder and going backward. A feeling of confusion is likely to prevail when we lose control of the schedule.

Now let's get to the classical, more objective symptoms of an unmanaged appointment schedule.

1. Demand is greater than access, delaying the time it takes for patients to get an appointment.
2. Frequent double-booking of appointments occurs.
3. The practice has more than an occasional no-show or late cancellation.
4. Patients experience long wait times once they arrive in the office.
5. Physicians get out of the office late, both mid-day and in the evening.
6. Charting is incomplete at the end of the day.
7. Staff continually work overtime.

If you recognize these symptoms, your scheduling patterns are *not* sensible. The scheduling system needs modification—in fact, it may need a complete overhaul.

Examine Scheduling Patterns

Take a look at the scheduling history to identify the factors that prevent a sensible schedule. Gather up appointment schedules for two weeks and take a critical look at how your day works.

The best way to predict future demand is to look at past demand and scheduling trends. Examine production patterns: how many patients are seen each day, the average number of patients seen per day, and the degree of disparity between the lowest- and highest-volume days for this two-week period. If you see more than a 20% variable on either side of the average, some strategic actions should be taken to improve this.

A second important component to examining scheduling demands is identifying the number of patients who are double-booked. How many patients you double-book or "squeeze in" indicates the needed capacity. Planning to meet this need will result in a better-managed schedule. After all, you are already seeing these patients, but most likely in a haphazard manner that results in delays and work left undone at the end of the day.

Document the Day

Next, gather data for a few days on the amount of time spent with each patient. This will help determine whether you are allotting enough time for each visit.

Table 1 offers a method for maintaining a time diary during the day. If Mr. Winterbug was scheduled simultaneously with Mrs. Feelgood, he could have been roomed quicker and his visit could have been accomplished without delaying care for Mrs. Feelgood. Dr. Efficient would have had both visits completed around 10:00 a.m. and would been able to start the visit with Mr. Meaniac sooner. It also may have been predictable that Mr. Meaniac would need more visit time, considering the multiple complaints that were not listed on the reason for the visit, and therefore should not be double-booked. In this case, double booking the 9:00 a.m. appointment would have been wiser than doubling up at 9:15. By 10:30 in the morning, Dr. Efficient was non-efficient and almost an hour behind schedule when Mr. Meaniac was finally seen.

TABLE 1. Appointment Time Study

Dr. Efficient / Monday, May 12th

Patient/appt time	Visit Reason	Patient Roomed	Doctor In	Doctor Out	Patient Room Out	Total Doctor Time (min.)
S. Feelgood/9:00	Annual physical	9:10	9:22	9:52	9:55	30
Comments: Required 10 min. prep time before Dr. could see patient.						
T. Winterbug/9:15	Cough	9:17	9:57	10:07	10:09	10
Comments: Tried to catch MD to see this patient before the annual physical						
J. Meaniac/9:15	Lethargic	9: 25	10:11	10:31	10:39	20
Comments: Patient upset at wait and had multiple medical complaints						
R. Niceguy/9:30	Swollen, painful finger	9:57	10:32	10:41	10:41	9
Comments: None						

The appointment time study helps indicate where problems occur and how they might have been avoided. It's a proactive way to examine how effectively you manage the daily schedule and identify what actions might help.

Another key to examining the day is to determine how many missed appointments occur each day. These cost you both time and money. If the average charge per patient encounter is $150 and there are three missed appointments a day, the practice is losing up to $30,000 a year in revenue.

This is even more costly when you consider the staff time involved in the process. For each missed appointment, time is required to schedule the appointment, pull the chart, document the no-show, and call the patient back—all for a patient who didn't generate revenue for the practice!

The missed appointment can compromise access as well. I've been in a number of practices where patients calling for appointments are required to wait an unrealistic amount of time for an appointment, or the physician resorts to telephone medicine (for which he is not paid), because "the schedule is full." In other words, we don't give the patient an appointment because we are holding it for a patient who isn't going to come in. Survey the patients who have missed appointments over the past thirty days and find out why, so you can do something about it. Typical reasons may be that:

- The patient was feeling better.
- The appointment was made so far out the patient forgot about it or decided to go elsewhere.
- The patient didn't think he would be missed.
- The patient didn't think it was important.

GET TO THE FIX

You've gathered all this information. Now what? Analyze the data and explore reasonable long-term solutions. Of course this requires a commitment—a commitment to change past habits and work diligently to develop a sensible schedule that will meet the specific needs of the practice and take you into the future.

Demand Versus Capacity

To establish a sensible schedule, match demand with capacity. Let's say your analysis reveals that the physician typically sees twenty-eight patients a day, even though there are only twenty-four slots. In other words, we need time to see four more patients each day. The physician, the scheduler, and the nurse can decide the best place is to add these patients to the schedule.

A modified wave schedule may suit your needs; this means scheduling two patients first thing in the morning and again in the afternoon. Patient selection is important for this to work. For example, a patient who requires a preliminary work-up or disrobing can be prepared for her visit while another patient requiring minimal preparation is being seen. You may want to use this same approach to create an additional slot mid-morning and mid-afternoon. This would provide the four slots that are needed to meet current demand. Keep in mind, high-intensity patients should not be double-booked in this fashion. The unpredictable time needs of these patients already make it difficult to stay on schedule. The effectiveness of a modified wave schedule really depends on the time of day when the physician finds she is the most efficient with her time and has the fewest interruptions.

The modified wave is just one approach to meeting demand. It might not be the right remedy for your practice style. Another approach is to change the amount of time allocated for each visit based on patient type. This may mean shifting from the typical fifteen-minute slot to ten-minute segments, allowing for more flexibility. Being realistic in determining the time needed for various types of patients will inevitably result in a more sensible schedule. For example, you may need three segments (30 minutes) for annual exams, but 20 minutes for camp physicals, and only one ten-minute segment for a follow-up on medications. At the same time, don't get too creative. Keep the various appointment types to less than five or you will be adding confusion that jeopardizes the entire concept. The appointment time study will be helpful in determining what is likely to work best.

Adopting an open access schedule is another way to meet scheduling demands, and it has become quite popular in the last few years. Open access schedules reserve a portion of the daily appointment schedule for same-day appointments, based on assumed demands. The assumptions are drawn by determining the average number of patients worked into the schedule in the past. Reserve this number of time slots on the appointment schedule, releasing them at a specific time, say the morning of the same day or at 4:00 p.m. the previous day. For example, if the magic number is ten added patients each day, and the practice dedicates fifteen minutes to each patient, it would be necessary to block out two and one-half hours each day for same-day appointments, perhaps one hour in the morning and one and one-half hours in the afternoon. This requires developing a new scheduling template that holds these appointments until the designated release time. The effective implementation date will depend on how far out you are currently booked. Once this type of schedule is implemented, some adjustments in the number of appointment slots may be required if the demand is greater or less during certain times of the year.

Should You Be a Groupie?

Group visits are a great way to work smarter instead of harder, but it takes some medical professionals outside their comfort zone. Most of us have a tendency to protect our existing methods of doing things. After all, there's a reason we do things the way we do—right? All the same, examining what is and isn't working will lead us to progressive thinking and opportunities to improve the way we work. When demand exceeds capacity, it makes sense to look at scheduling alternatives.

In some instances, group visits are very effective. They improve access and efficiency while giving collections a boost. They're an attractive method of treating and managing patients with similar needs, such as post-operative joint replacement or childbirth classes. And they offer these patients the opportunity to interact, gain support, and learn from each other.

Group visits are an effective technique to help manage chronic illnesses such as diabetes and hypertension, for which patients need extensive instructions, education, and support. The group visit models are designed to improve patient satisfaction, quality of life, and quality of care. Because patients are managed in a group setting, access improves, as well as patient compliance, leading to reduced emergency room visits and potentially better outcomes. Sounds like a win–win to me.

After implementing shared medical appointments, the Palo Alto Medical Clinic in California reported a 200%–300% increase in productivity while improving access[1], the bottom line, and both patient and physician satisfaction.

The fundamental reason group visits work is that a relatively small portion of the appointment time is dedicated to the actual exam. The remainder of the session, typically sixty to ninety minutes, is spent on the interactive component of the exam: educating the patients, discussing self-management, providing peer support, and transforming their commitment to better health.

There are some logistic challenges involved with group visits. You must have an available conference room in close proximity to a private room for the individual exams, which typically take six to nine minutes per patient. Managing the patient flow and wait time can require some finesse, as can insuring the appropriate levels of confidentiality and privacy. You must be cognizant of HIPAA regulations and require each patient to sign a confidentiality statement. It's also important to monitor the drop-out rate, which tends to be low for weekly visits and high for three- to six-month intervals.

The success of group visits relies on advanced planning, the use of professional resources for education and support, and having a good facilitator who understands group dynamics and can effectively control and manage the interactive session. Managing group visits takes a team and requires cooperation at different levels.

Managing Missed Appointments

It's important to confirm appointments to let patients know you expect them to be there and to hold them accountable. Refer to these as appointment confir-

---

[1] Noffsinger, Edward. "Physicals Shared Medical Appointments: A Revolutionary Access Solution," *Group Practice Journal*, January 2002, 51(1).

mations instead of reminders; this distinction puts the responsibility of keeping the appointment on the patient. At the same time, make sure the staff does not give patients subtle messages that imply the appointment is not important.

Whether appointment reminders are automated or manual, choose your words carefully. Some verbiage actually guides a patient to assuming the appointment is not important or that they have permission to cancel. Saying "Let us know if you can't keep your 3:30 appointment," gives the patient permission to cancel. It is far better to say, "Dr. Well is expecting you at 3:30." And "I'm squeezing you in at 11," makes the patient think he will be waiting a long time or that he won't be missed if he doesn't show up. "Doctor can see you for an 11 a.m. appointment" tells the patient you are dedicating time just for him. It's amazing how you can shift the attitude of the patients and make an immediate impact on the missed appointment rate.

Technology is now available to manage patient reminders at a fraction of the costs to do it manually. These systems are reliable, reinforce the importance of the appointment, reduce the missed appointment rate, and provide an accurate record of patients who were contacted and when.

Of course, if you want patients to value your time, you must value theirs— and that means *staying on schedule and on time!*

GAIN AN EDGE ON TIME

Think creatively when looking for scheduling solutions—how to maximize existing resources and space. The goal is to help the physician maximize efficiency as she works her way through the schedule. That means having the right tools, including well-equipped rooms, well-trained support staff, and ways to minimize interruptions and reduce steps. Consider all of these factors when developing a sensible schedule. It's about freeing up physician time around the visit—time taken up with tasks that do not require her expertise. These tasks may be essential, but someone else can be doing them so the physician's time is spent with the patient and the quality of the visit is better for everyone . . . most importantly the patient!

Staying on Time

The trick to staying on time is a sensible schedule that both honors the appointment and makes the most of the time dedicated to the appointment schedule. When support staff perceives the physician (and visit) needs, the physician makes better use of his time. The time span between the patient's arrival and the physician entering the room is a critical factor to making the best use of time and managing the schedule.

If there is something that can be done for the visit before the patient is seen by the physician, staff needs to do this in advance. Without exception this includes the following tasks.

1. Charts properly prepared: Make sure the patient's medical record is current. This includes all diagnostic studies available, updated medications list, current problem list, and anything else the physicians in your practice need to understand the patient's current health status.

2. Tending to preliminary visit activities: If a follow-up lab, EKG, urinalysis, or other studies are expected, have these completed before the patient is seen by the physician.

3. Rooming the patient: Develop a matrix for preparing patients for the visit and keep it either at the nursing station or in each exam room. This matrix should include what needs to occur before the patient is seen by the physician. Does the patient need to disrobe? Do you need to get a weight and height, take vitals, etc.?

4. Obtaining a proper clinical history: The nurse can save the physician time by getting a more detailed clinical history. For example, if Mrs. Smith has a cough and fever, how long has she had it? Is she coughing up mucous? Is there a loss of appetite or a fever? How long have these symptoms existed?

5. Perceiving the physician's needs and meeting them beforehand: Clinical staff can learn to predict what the physician may need during the visit. For example, if the patient has fluid on the knee, why not set up for a needle aspiration before the doctor ever enters the room? Having bandages ready for the patient that is a vein stripping post-op is another example. Whatever your specialty, there are certain patients for whom some of the clinical actions and the requirements to accomplish them are predictable. When staff tends to these needs in advance, the physician works swiftly and will not need to come in and out of the exam room during the visit to get these needs met.

With a little effort, physicians can train their clinical staff to perform these types of tasks the way they want them done and ensure that the quality of outcomes is not compromised. By doing so you not only save time, you enrich office roles. It supports camaraderie, makes employees' contributions more meaningful and increases accountability. In the end, it creates consistency and reliability in managing the schedule. You can see there is a lot to be gained, including staying on time!

Creating the right schedule requires thoughtful planning and a clear understanding of why a well-managed schedule has eluded you in the past. Examining historical patterns, predicting scheduling needs (both demand and time), understanding how you work, and knowing what actions will contribute to improved efficiency provide an effective approach to achieving the coveted sensible schedule. ●

TAKE BACK TIME

- *Study the indicators that represent an unmanaged schedule.*
- *Existing scheduling patterns predict patient scheduling needs.*
- *Take a critical look at how you manage the daily schedule.*
- *Capacity and demands must intersect to create a sensible schedule.*
- *Missed appointments cost the practice time and money.*
- *Effective use of support staff is an essential ingredient to getting an edge on time.*

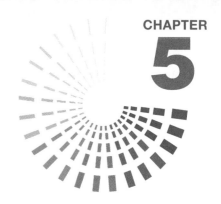

Get It Right!

"Quality is never an accident; it is always the result of high intention, sincere effort, intelligent direction, and skillful execution."

—*Willa A. Foster*

When I first envisioned writing a book to help healthcare profession-als with managing the enormous demands on their time, I knew there would be a chapter devoted to quality. Understanding how the variables in quality impact the use of time offers a convincing reason to focus on quality. Quality needs to be a priority throughout healthcare delivery systems, even without the pressures of outside forces.

As defined in the dictionary, quality is a "degree of excellence." (*New World Dictionary*) Achieving and maintaining a high degree of excellence will result in greater efficiency and that precious commodity, time. Obtaining and maintaining impressive quality results within the practice requires a commitment. The commitment is not an edict that is given to someone. It is setting the goal and taking actions to achieve it. Those actions must include establishing specific measurable indicators, monitoring performance, and holding physicians and staff accountable to achieve a pre-set mark.

You may get the feeling quality is a fad. We all remember when total quality management, TQM, became the rage in organizational management in the late 1990s. TQM focuses on managing and continuously *improving* quality. It moves beyond quality assurance, which may seek only to inspect and correct errors to achieve a reliable outcome.

In recent years quality theories have again come to forefront as Six Sigma, a system designed to improve processes and eliminate defects, has gotten the attention of businesses seeking to improve quality by applying sound quality management principles to reduce variations in process and achieve better outcomes. Medical practices can no longer ignore this information as only applicable to big business—it applies to all businesses, and a medical practice is a business!

The emphasis on quality is striving to "get it right" the first time. That's a lofty goal. It's also somewhat unrealistic, as it implies we don't make mistakes. Everyone knows we make mistakes, and the resulting lessons lead to improved processes and better solutions, bringing us closer to the perfection we strive to attain. Our odds of getting it right improve when we're on a quest for quality.

Errors are most expected during two different scenarios: training and monitoring change. Improving the outcome in these scenarios requires closely monitoring performance and giving prompt feedback and encouragement.

Training

We expect that a new employee, and/or existing employee who is learning a new skill is bound to experience a learning curve that involves an occasional error before achieving proficiency. The responsibility of determining an acceptable error ratio belongs to management. For this reason it is incredibly important to dedicate time to train employees properly and reduce variations in how a task is accomplished. We must also communicate our expectations during the training period. Because the learning curve varies with individuals, it is essential to closely monitor the consistency and overall performance of each new employee. Not only do we discover where the employee needs help, we give them support, increase their skills and confidence, help them strive to reach our expectations, and help them to avoid costly errors in the future.

Managing change

When changes are implemented people may have a knee-jerk reaction and perform tasks the "old way." Sometimes staff will fail to listen due to an unintentional resistance to change. As a result they lack an understanding of what is expected and what is required to succeed, which can compromise a quality result. Inevitably, a step or two is missed, resulting in errors.

MAKE QUALITY A PRIORITY

We are challenged to make quality a priority in how we deliver healthcare. Government, payers, and the public are all focused on quality. Medical and administrative errors contribute to the high cost of healthcare, and like it or not, put you and your practice under the microscope when it comes to examining quality.

Indicators of Poor Quality

Poor outcomes will inevitably lead to compromised finances, increased emotional distress, patient dissatisfaction, inconsistency, and poor use of time. To gain a clearer understanding of the cost of poor quality, let's review some specific indicators. We'll see that each of these can be costly to both time and finances.

Inspection and Rework Costs

Think of the responsibility of generating an insurance claim. If it's done right the first time, you get paid quickly and the employee is on to other tasks. If it is rejected, the employee must do additional work to inspect and rework the claim, and the employer must invest in further training to reduce the potential for errors to continue. Several questions emerge: what error was made, why or how did it happen, and how can it be fixed for the long-term?

Overstaffing

Inconsistent and poor outcomes result in extra steps and more time. It begins with the time required to put out the fires (crisis management). Something as simple as taking and responding to a phone message becomes time-consuming when it isn't done right. If the message is incomplete or the phone number is wrong, a number of steps and time are required to fix the problem, even before you decide how to handle the message and reach final disposition. It takes additional staff to fix errors and keep the work flowing, so you end up overstaffing to fix recurring problems, rather than intervening in a way that eliminates the potential for this error to reappear.

Long waiting times

If we aren't managing the schedule well, how can we manage the day? The challenges become obvious. Patients will be delayed, and physicians and staff will not leave the office on time. When this happens, you pay dearly. The costs go up, but the revenue declines. The problem stems from poor performance and mismanagement.

Disintegrating work environment

Think about the impressions you get when you cannot depend on the quality you will receive at a store or business. I remember switching to a different drug store chain because I experienced pricing errors over and over due to incorrect scanning, because the staff failed to update pricing on the scanner. That meant I had to watch every item I purchased, knowing one out of ten would be wrong. Then the checker would need to call someone over to ask about it, and someone else needed to do a price-check. This resulted in a lack of trust on my part, and because I could not depend on being charged correctly, I no longer patronized that store.

The drug store incurs other costs for the irregularity in scanning prices. It creates a bottleneck at the check-out counter as customers back up, wasting time for both the consumer and the employee. Add to this the financial cost for all this inefficiency and you get the picture. Think about something similar happening in your practice—it would erode profits, confuse staff, and result in customer frustration and lack of confidence.

Disgruntled Patients and Staff

It can happen to you! Staff attitudes affect the quality of services and outcomes. If patients experience inconsistency in the way you deliver either business or clinical outcomes, they will feel compromised and confused. Since many inconsistencies result from a lack of well-defined processes and accountability, staff will believe there is nothing they can do about it. Their disenchantment will inevitably lead to poor morale, compromised service, and higher staff turnover.

Lost Market Share

As exhibited in the example of the drug store scanners, patients who feel they cannot depend on you will go elsewhere for their care. If you are a specialist, you can bet unhappy patients will report their dissatisfaction to their primary care physicians, and future referrals may decline. This can quickly erode the stability of a practice.

Lower Profits

The steps and costs required to continually fix problems, correct errors, and live with redundancies scream out for attention. The investment of time and other resources to streamline processes and develop consistent quality outcomes is essential to the future of healthcare providers. When physicians and management are not committed to quality, the practice is being short-sighted.

Quality has too often remained an ill-defined, intangible object. In reality, achieving quality begins with a commitment that is proven by the actions taken to deliberately measure specific outcomes and determine what variables can be altered to provide a more predictable and satisfactory outcome.

The Cost of Poor Quality

It becomes very clear that the high cost of poor quality lies in correcting errors. Knowing where the majority of errors occur in the delivery of healthcare is quite revealing. A study conducted by American Academy of Family Physicians[1], shows that 66% of medical errors with primary care physicians are a direct result of process problems (34%) and charting errors (32%). Additional causes for medical errors included, "ordered care not provided" (15%), "medication error" (13%), "clinical judgment" (3%) and "inter-specialty communication" (3%). These high percentages for process problems and charting errors provide a powerful reason to intervene and take corrective action. These errors are very costly to the consumer, the payer, and the practice. By developing consistent, reliable processes and having providers chart in real time, these medical errors would be reduced.

LOST IN TIME: A CLASSIC CASE STUDY

Help Needed Group Practice was drowning. They had classic symptoms of being in troubled waters, and the practice was out of control.

- Excessive time spent looking for charts
- Repeat phone calls
- Angry patients
- Long hours and overtime
- Delay in patient care
- Patient attrition
- Employee turnover

A review of practice operations revealed that standard processes did not exist for many primary tasks, including time allotted for each appointment, information required to complete a telephone intake, time parameters and legibility for chart documentation, patient rooming, and exam room stocking. There was no feedback mechanism to monitor patient satisfaction or to register a complaint and make sure it was resolved to the patient's (and practice's) satisfaction. Employee performance evaluations were not tied to specific, objective performance standards. This resulted in confusion and a lot of lost time. Thus practice had a choice; value everyone's time by standardizing procedures and increasing accountability or add more staff to support the inefficiencies. Help Needed recognized the time and customer service gains they would experience by eliminating variations in how work is done and holding everyone accountable to a specific standard.

---

[1] Monitor, "The Root of Primary Care Errors," *Family Practice Management*, American Academy of Family Physicians, February 2001.

Most practices know when inefficiencies exist; they experience the cause and effect. But here's a simple test that lets you know it's time to take corrective steps.

The Twelve-Point Inefficiency Test

1. Staff works late.
2. Today's work is *not* completed at the end of the day (charting/dictation, posting charges, receipts and adjustments, filing).
3. Claims are more than occasionally rejected because of incomplete or inaccurate information.
4. The accounts receivable over ninety days is more than 25% of the total accounts receivable.
5. Patients complain about being kept on hold.
6. We get more than an occasional repeat caller during the day (someone that called earlier and is calling back for the same reason).
7. The average patient wait in the reception room is more than fifteen minutes.
8. Physicians get interrupted in the exam room.
9. Physicians do not come into the office on time.
10. The office is running a parallel medical record system more than six months after implementing electronic medical records.
11. We run out of supplies.
12. Performance reviews are overdue.

"Yes" answers to these questions indicate inefficient or inconsistent outcomes. Your practice needs to take a hard look at how things are being done and the amount of time that is wasted due to delays, errors, and inconsistencies.

The rest of this chapter will define ways a practice can resolve the typical quality issues that compromise performance and satisfaction for patients, staff, and physicians.

THE LEAN MACHINE

Some practices are aware of the different steps that are repeated and compromise efficiency, while others just struggle to keep up with the workload, never taking time to develop shortcuts that will make the job easier. The highly efficient practice is within your reach if you are willing to examine processes and eliminate redundancy and waste. It takes a "lean machine" to make the most of resources and deliver consistent quality outcomes.

Creating the lean machine begins with a very important concept: identify the steps that add value to practice operations and patient service, and eliminate those that are unnecessary. To accomplish this you need to carefully examine the details of how tasks are completed. Ask yourself why these steps are taken and whether there is a more efficient way to accomplish the end result.

Certainly with the advent of new technologies, we can remove a number of manual processes, and in so doing, create fewer variations in outcomes. This means involving the people that do the work; based on their knowledge and your guidance, new lean work flow designs can be integrated to improve efficiency. This is true for both clinical and business performance measures.

Cut Steps

Effectively cutting steps requires a careful examination of current practices:
- What main steps are currently in place?
- How do *people* move through the process?
- How does *information* move through the process?
- What are the critical points of variation?
- Where is the value?
- What is wasteful, redundant, or simply unnecessary?

You are likely to be amazed at where the waste is. It might be a system that double-checks and triple-checks work, a process that corrects errors made by someone who simply needs proper training, or a "that's the way we've always done it" mentality that uses manual processes that can be automated to save steps and time and improve consistency.

Let's look at some potential work problems that eat away at the typical practice's time and compromise patient service. When you look at Table 1, think about the number of steps that are reduced by the solution, the time that is saved, and the consistency that is gained.

Reduce Variations

Now it's time to get leaner by reducing those variations. Create a flow chart that defines the main steps of the procedure as they have been done in the past. Then move on to determine what steps can be eliminated and what refined steps will result in improved efficiency. This is not a one-person

TABLE 1. Improving Work Flow

Problem	Example	Solution
Work interruption	Receptionist leaving work station to photocopy patient insurance card	Place card scanner at receptionist work station.
Unbalanced workload	Billing department inundated with patient phone calls first week of each month	1. Cycle bill patient statements by sending a particular alphabetical section each week. 2. Improve patient dunning messages. 3. Implement a patient-friendly, easy-to-understand billing statement.
Poor planning	Running out of essential medical supplies	Develop an inventory tracking system that notifies you when supplies are low.
Inconsistent patient compliance	Fair percentage of target female patients not being scheduled for mammograms	Implement an automated reminder system with a built-in tracking tool.
Performing tasks that do not add value	Extensive manual processes to create bank deposit, make the deposit, and file and retrieve EOBs	Secure a bank lock box for mail-in payments. Bank will electronically mail you a copy of the checks, EOBs, and deposit. EOBs are stored electronically.
Provider interruption	Leaving exam room because of missing consult, lab, or diagnostic reports	Develop a pre-visit process and chart preparation that includes reviewing/auditing chart notes and reports generated from the previous visit.
Fluctuating variations in demand	High demand for pre-kindergarten physicals and inoculations in August	Send reminders in May for patients to schedule throughout the summer.

show; it must involve the people who do the work. Their knowledge and experiences will ensure each step in the process is included in the flow chart. With leadership's guidance, more efficient, lean processes will emerge and help raise the quality bar.

Have a Quality Plan

A quality commitment starts at the top and must hold both physicians and staff accountable. To develop a quality plan that makes sense for your organization, define your values and desired outcomes.

TABLE 2. Sample Quality Plan Matrix—Gynecology Practice

Area of focus	Performance Measure	Goal	Value
Employee Satisfaction	Timely performance evaluations	Accomplish within ten days of anniversary of hire	Improved employee morale, better communication, higher performance
Patient Satisfaction	Reduced wait time for patients	Decrease average wait time from twenty-five minutes to ten minutes by (goal date)	Improved patient experience, increased practice efficiency, and decreased overtime costs
Clinical Performance	Improved compliance with annual pap smear	At least 95% of appropriate patients pre-scheduled for annual exam and pap. Each patient will receive phone and/or e-mail confirmation within forty-eight hours of scheduled appointment.	Improved patient care and compliance
Business Performance	Accurate patient demographics/insurance information	Less than 2% of claims rejected based on demographics/insurance information	Improved time management, profitability, and cash flow

It is best to explore business performance, clinical performance, and both patient and staff satisfaction, and then select measures that will improve results in these primary areas. These measures should be selected based on areas of sub-par performance in the past. Check out the examples in Table 2.

PAY FOR PERFORMANCE

Many physicians are both concerned and confused about all the discussion on pay for performance, P4P. There are plenty of unknowns on where the research and focus on quality measures will lead. One thing is apparent: government and other third-party payers are looking at ways to tie performance to the amount they pay for healthcare services as a means to control the continuing rise in healthcare costs.

The primary emphasis on performance is identifying measures that will ensure improvement and consistency in patient safety, quality of care, and patient satisfaction. The objective is to improve the standard of care while reducing inefficiencies that contribute to a continued rise in healthcare costs. It's not a matter of one shoe fits all, but rather a matter of recognizing these key elements of practice performance and examining how you might address them within your own practice.

Most of the pilot programs underway are designed to measure processes and identify how often physicians provide appropriate treatments or tests. The goal is to address quality issues and improve outcomes.

The emerging programs focus on three primary elements:

1. Patient satisfaction
2. Adoption of computer technology
3. Effective clinical treatment and preventive measures

It is my hope that physicians will respond thoughtfully to future P4P initiatives. It would be wise to examine variables in practice performance related to patient service and care. Within that realm, think about the patient experience and the inconsistencies that exist in your office.

Access is a good example since it affects both patient satisfaction and clinical outcomes. The longer patients wait to be seen, the greater the likelihood that their conditions may worsen. Look to see how far ahead a patient must book to get the next available appointment. Does it realistically meet the patients' needs, and is it consistent among the providers? For example, does a patient wait three weeks to see Dr. A when Dr. C can see him within five days? If so, it would not take long for Dr. A's patients to feel short-changed and want to shift to another physician in the group or leave the practice.

Don't assume patients are satisfied with the care and services you offer— ask them! There are a number of ways to do this.

- Patient satisfaction surveys
- Focus groups
- New patient post-encounter interview
- Mystery patient visits

A critical component to gathering patient satisfaction results is a willingness to address and fix problems that are identified.

One of the primary factors in implementing clinical outcome measures is physician agreement. The physicians must know, understand, and agree on what to measure and how it will be measured.

Select an indicator that is clinically significant for which the data is not too difficult to obtain. An example for urology might be looking at how consistently the practice orders prostate specific antigen (PSA) testing to screen for prostate cancer.

1. Is a PSA ordered every three years or every five years?
2. At what age do you begin, and is it consistent among the providers?
3. How do you monitor compliance?

In other words, do the physicians agree on a standard? Do they apply the standard consistently, and are your methods of monitoring compliance effective? If the physicians disagree, there are a number of ways to reach consensus.

- Gather objective data that supports each physician's rationale for his specific recommendation.
- Turn to the appropriate specialty academy or association for a recommended clinical pathway.
- Conduct peer review sessions and clinical audits to assess practice outcomes.

In reality physicians have always been paid for their performance. The more efficient they are and the better they manage costs, the better the bottom line. The difference in the future will be in how third–party payers reimburse a practice. It is expected that some payers will pay as much as a 10% premium differential for top-performing practices. Most physicians will find the potential for revenue gains of $50,000 to $100,000 a significant incentive to get on board with P4P.

There are plenty of reasons to implement programs that measure quality and intervene when performance can be improved. Keep in mind that the ultimate goal with P4P is to improve the health of your patients and the health of the practice. By being proactive, you can do it your way, with a meaningful approach that focuses on what is important to you and your patients.

Quality programs also need to tie individual staff performance to specific quality measures. This begins with defining quality processes in the job description, performance standards, and the performance evaluation. It then becomes a pay-for-quality-performance issue for each employee and management.

---

[2] Dahl, O. *Think Business! Medical Practice Quality, Efficiency, Profits*, Phoenix, Md., Greenbranch Publishing, 2007, page 43. www.mpmnetwork.com

So how committed are you to quality? My friend Owen Dahl[2] challenges the healthcare profession by asking, "What is the question most often heard in the practice? Is it what was today's deposit, or is it what was today's quality score?" ⬤

TAKE BACK TIME
- *Mistakes lead to improved processes and better solutions.*
- *Focus on training and managing change results in reducing errors.*
- *Poor quality wastes time and resources.*
- *Creating a lean machine and improving work flow design requires involving the people who do the work.*
- *Employee knowledge and experience, coupled with management's guidance, bring better results.*
- *Cutting steps and reducing variations save time and improve outcomes.*
- *Committing to quality includes developing a quality plan that makes sense to the organization improving patient and staff satisfaction, clinical outcomes and business performance.*
- *Employee job expectations and performance should include quality measures.*

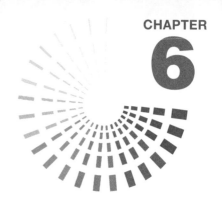

CHAPTER

6

Make the Most of Staff

"Life is just a mirror and what you see out there, you must first see inside of you."

—Wally "Famous" Amos

THE "YOU'RE GREAT" CULTURE

L eadership sets the tone for staff's performance and how well the people that work with you utilize their time. It starts with you. Employees will mirror your behavior. So if you set the example, they will learn to be prudent with both time and resources. If you create an environment that makes staff feel important and appreciated, you will be amazed at what they will accomplish for you. It's the "you're great" culture that results in a spirit of cooperation, staff taking ownership of the practice, and everyone in the practice being committed to top performance and the best use of time. A word of caution—telling staff they're great won't cut it. Talk's cheap! It is leadership's attitude and actions that will either make them feel valued, or quite the opposite, think you simply don't care.

The "BE" Attitudes

Here's my list of BE attitudes and how to apply them for a "you're great" culture.

BElieve

The dictionary's definition of believe is "to accept as true or real." (*New World Dictionary*) So ask yourself: "Do I believe the staff is outstanding, striving to be their best, and that each person feels the practice is his responsibility, as well as mine?" Wow! That's a lot to expect of staff, and in many years consulting with medical practices, I can tell you it is rare. Just the same, it is achievable.

It starts by getting in touch with staff so you understand them better. Make no assumptions about how they feel about their jobs; find out. And let them make no assumptions about what you expect from them or how much you appreciate them. Communicate your expectations and make sure employees agree that these expectations are realistic. Quantify and qualify the expectation: "Laura, we want to see the aged receivables over ninety days reduced to under 20% of the total A/R by the end of the first quarter. What can I do to help your department achieve this?" Now the ball is in Laura's court, and it's up to her to communicate her department's needs to reach the expectation. If she doesn't think your expectations are realistic, you can either adjust the expectation or help her develop a plan to achieve it.

Be consistent, fair, and sincere. Give staff an opportunity to expand their skills, taking on more responsibility and accomplishing more—and remember to acknowledge a job well done!

BE Visible

When physicians and managers are not accessible and visible to staff on a daily basis, there is an unspoken barrier between them and the people they depend on, their staff. Optimal performance and wise use of time require a team that is inspired by the example they see. Say good morning to everyone, walk through the facility every chance you get, and make efforts to interact with people in each department, at various levels. The simple things you do that express appreciation and show respect make the difference. Treat everyone the same, whether it's a manager or the file clerk. Your visibility will result in employees emulating your actions. That's powerful!

BE Supportive

Managing employees is a challenge, especially when today's healthcare professionals have so much on their plates. One more employee problem looks like it will keep you from getting to the work that needs your attention. In reality, if you support staff and help them to grow their skills, the time investment will result in employees' confidence increasing to a level that they will be able to self-manage and depend on you less. At the same time they will know when something needs your attention and when it's time to involve you. This has the potential to save you a great deal of time and keep employees more productive.

I was once in a practice where the administrator believed so strongly in his employees that he knew if he was absent the work would go on without skipping a beat. I asked him how often he called the practice if he was out of the office attending a conference for, say, four to five days. He confidently said, "I never call the practice. Why would I? They can handle most day-to-day activities, and if they know something needs my attention they will call or e-mail." I thought that was wonderful and went on to ask him how often that happened. He assured me it was rare, because his employees were great. He has the magic formula when it comes to supporting and cultivating employees.

BE Timely

I've covered timeliness in other areas of this book; now I'll review what it means to your employees when you make time a priority. Many of you are thinking, "Oh yeah, we need to put time parameters on employees and hold them accountable." Well, this is true. But when it comes to giving employees the "you're great" message, I'm referring to how well you keep your promises when it comes to meeting deadlines that affect employees. Failing to do this jeopardizes the confidence staff have in you and their willingness to go the extra mile for the practice.

Several areas represent a call to action when it comes to being timely, making employees feel important, and maintaining both morale and productivity. Don't postpone or delay these important activities:

● Staff meetings.
● Employee performance reviews.
● Staff reports, such as an employee reporting at a staff meeting on information learned at a recent continuing medical education forum.
● Celebrated events, such as the annual office picnic, Christmas, or holiday party.
● Cost of living pay increases.
● Authorizations of requested time off.
● Employee training.

Calendar these events well in advance. Once you commit to these scheduled activities, recognize the impact that keeping this schedule has on staff and how they feel valued. Honor time—theirs and yours!

BUILD ON THEIR STRENGTHS

The coach is, without question, a leader that motivates people and builds them up with a "you can do it" attitude. Just as importantly, the coach is a management diagnostician that can develop a treatment plan to improve confidence, commitment, and performance for both individuals and groups. Here are a few ideas on how to apply your coaching skills and build on staff strengths.

What Makes Them Tick?

Getting inside the heads of your employees is a major challenge, but doing so enables you to help them be more productive and use time wisely. You deal with many personalities, and it's your job to find out not only what motivates them, but what type of worker each one is. By doing so, you will be able to build on individual strengths to improve their personal satisfaction, their confidence, and team performance. The results can be incredible. Make a list for each employee with two columns, one that describes his or her motivators, and one that describes the type of worker he or she is.

Motivators

You probably have an idea of what the key motivators are for each employee, so list them out. Here are some typical motivators:

- Praise
- Recognition
- Social status
- Flexibility
- Responsibility
- Challenge
- Money
- Professional growth

Once you have listed your initial thoughts on paper for each individual, you can refine the list. Gain clarity by meeting with each employee to discuss the things that excite him about his work and what he finds challenging. This will help clarify the accuracy of your impressions. The employee's contribution to this is key to reaching a clear understanding of what the employee values. The project can prove to be an interesting assignment that is insightful and may even reveal some unexpected end results.

Worker Type

By worker type, I am referring to the traits of the individual in relationship to her work performance. For example, some people are multi-taskers, juggling many tasks simultaneously and getting each one accomplished efficiently. Other people are more linear and can be great taskmasters, focusing on one assignment at a time. Then there are the independent workers who do their best when they fly solo rather than sharing work to accomplish the same end result. Each worker type makes a valuable contribution to the practice, and that value increases when managers know how to tap into these traits. When assigning job responsibilities, focus on the individuals and how each one spends her time. This keeps employees challenged and productive, contributes to greater efficiency, and ultimately leads to better time management.

Fast-track learning

Not so long ago, providing continuing education opportunities for staff involved sending employees to a conference outside the office where they attended a workshop or lecture. Such sessions are valuable and create an opportunity to network and learn from others. However, they require a lot of time out of the office and represent an element of downtime as staff members travel to and from these sessions. New educational opportunities bring the sessions to the employees. I call this fast-track learning.

Lunch and Learn

Lunch and learn programs offer a number of advantages. They allow information to be brought to the entire staff in an efficient way, right on the job. It can be a matter of closing the office for two hours over lunch and having a session in the staff lounge or the reception area. There are a number of ways to accomplish this:

1. Bring in a live speaker on the topic of your choice.
2. Host webinars, for which a speaker provides distance learning through a PowerPoint presentation.
3. Participate in audio conferences that permit the entire staff to "attend" for one fee, and for which you can download the presentation materials in advance.
4. Purchase educational audio books or lectures.

Distance Learning

Technology has definitely opened up this creative channel for learning, giving employees a way to obtain valuable certifications right from their desks. The distinguished Certified Medical Manager with the Professional Association of Health Care Office Management (PAHCOM) is just one example.

The Medical Group Management Association, MGMA, encourages its members to expand their knowledge through its core learning series. MGMA offers a broad range of online courses that enable medical practice leaders to obtain the American College of Medical Practice Executives certification. This designation has great value in the marketplace for medical practice administrators and executives.

The American College of Healthcare Executives, ACHE, also has expanded its credentialing program to include online courses to become a fellow, or

FACHE. Clearly, if you want to increase your knowledge and value in the market, you can do it online, saving lots of time.

Management can determine what investment to make to open up this door of opportunity. Some practices pay for the enrollment but expect the employee to take the course after hours. Others are willing to give the employee time to participate on the job. For organizations that make a substantial investment in upgrading skills, it is prudent to expect the employee to stay with the organization eighteen to twenty-four months afterwards. In order to accomplish this, explain your requirements up front. For example, you may expect the employee to absorb 75% of the costs if she resigns within the first eighteen months after the course, and 50% if she leaves between eighteen and twenty-four months afterward.

Think creatively when it comes to educational support for employees, individually or as a group. You might want to set aside time each month and have your own learning channel or internal educational book club, for example the third Wednesday of each month from 4:00 to 5:00 p.m. This supports professional growth and will make effective use of time.

To further support this philosophy, try implementing a "bring it back" program to make the most of it when a staff member attends an outside conference. As a stipulation to approving the activity, require the individual to bring back three learning points to share at the next staff meeting.

Stretch Their Limits

The more you expect from staff, the more they grow. The more they grow, the more they contribute. If you stretch employees to learn more and take on more responsibility, they will become more enthusiastic about their work. No longer will they feel like they are stuck in a rut or on the road to nowhere. This improves job performance and staff longevity, reducing the many hours and high costs required to recruit, select, hire, train, and integrate new staff.

Your success in stretching the limits of staff depends on your ability to analyze their individual potentials, recognize their strengths, identify growth opportunities, delegate effectively, and demonstrate sincere confidence in your staff's ability to take on new challenges.

CAN WE ALL GET ALONG?

I'll bet everyone that reads this book has a story or two they could tell about the negative impact on production that becomes clearly visible when staff members do not get along. It can be a major disaster that affects not only staff productivity, but your own as well.

Reduce Potential Conflict

Conflicts are bound to emerge. The office environment becomes much like a family and bickering just happens. At the same time, we look for ways to reduce it so people get back to work. I remember dealing with my own children when they were young and either finding ways to diffuse disagreements or separating them to keep minor incidents from erupting into major explosions that consumed my time and taxed my ability to cope. Many of you are thinking, "Been there, done that!" Those practical skills you learned in your personal life as a sibling, a friend, or a parent can serve you well in understanding ways to reduce work conflicts at an early stage.

Our practice team is our work family. Sometimes our staff becomes too comfortable, too sensitive, or too competitive to keep a realistic perspective. As leaders of the practice, we must find ways to reduce the potential for conflict by recognizing why the conflicts emerge in the first place.

Conflicts emerge for a variety of reasons. Individuals who work with you have different needs and objectives; they even have different beliefs and core values. Yet we must create a stimulating team environment in the workplace, which is easier said then done. Add to this turf battles and misconceptions, and the potential for conflict becomes evident.

Staff's perceptions rarely match management's. Employee issues and concerns are far different and at a more personal level. They want to feel and believe that everyone is doing their fair share. If Justin thinks he is working harder or has more problems than Dana, or if he even perceives he doesn't get the support he deserves, problems begin to fester. It becomes a "me against them" attitude. Think about it—wouldn't that put you on the offense in a hurry? The resentments build and the perceptions become reality. Once a member of your staff is resentful or becomes self-serving, you can bet a conflict is on the horizon.

Successfully avoiding conflict begins with a structure that clearly defines each person's role and responsibilities in the office, including how his position and actions support his peers. This means establishing clear lines of authority and responsibility, and developing realistic job descriptions that explain individual tasks. Eliminate the opportunity for staff to fall into the "it's not in my job description" trap by including a statement that the person will be responsible for "other duties, as assigned." When delivering a job description, communicate how each person's responsibilities support the others and contribute to reaching common goals for the practice. It is through this process that we build a strong, supportive team—the foundation for efficiency and higher levels of productivity.

Manage Conflict Better

To manage a conflict we must recognize that it is emerging and provide early intervention. It is likely to start with a minor complaint, but if the complaint is ignored, it festers and dissension grows. This is not to say that every complaint becomes a conflict that management must address.

Many issues are conflict-tolerant, meaning they are easily resolved between the parties involved or simply dissolve on their own. If Justin and Dana are having problems and can work it out on their own, so much the better. This is far more likely to happen if management provides an encouraging and supportive environment in which employees communicate in a healthy way and are tuned in to understanding other points of view.

When this doesn't work, management must intervene. Meet individually with Justin and Dana to listen to their take on the situation.

- Listen with all your senses to what's being said, how it's being said, what is unspoken, and visual cues that signal whether a cooperative spirit exists. Someone with arms crossed and failure to give eye contact clearly sends a far different message than someone with a relaxed posture and open arms, who is looking at you while they speak.
- Clarify what has been said: your interpretation versus their impressions.
- Gain a clear understanding of each person's perspective.

Now it's time to meet together with Justin and Dana. The goal is to bring objectivity to the table and facilitate a mutually agreeable solution. The emotions must be managed. This requires you to guide the discussion and stick with the facts, so it doesn't get personal. It may be necessary to run interference so Justin or Dana don't get off track and attack one another. By staying focused on the specifics they will learn to respect each other's point of view and work toward a resolution. It's a matter of focusing on the solution, rather than the problem. Following the discussion,

1. Clearly define the problem.
2. Identify and explain the options to resolve the problem.

3. Clarify questions or concerns related to the proposed options.

4. Agree on the solution and how it will be implemented.

Hopefully you can resolve conflicts the first time around. If not, set a deadline for resolution, provide guidance, and meet again as the deadline approaches. Setting a deadline holds everyone accountable to resolve the issues and get back to a healthy work environment. I am often amazed at how well management succeeds when they put the responsibility on the individuals, provide structure and guidance, and get out of the way. It can be done, and the sooner conflicts are addressed, the sooner we get back to people really getting along.

IT'S THE CAM

Most people want to be productive at work, but need leadership and structure to fulfill this goal so that they feel good about what they do each day. I see three basic issues that make the biggest difference in management getting the most out of employees and fully appreciating each person's contributions: communication, accountability, and motivation—CAM. It makes a world of difference in the team you develop and maintain.

Communication

Too often we assume someone knows what we are thinking and what we want from them. Too often we fail to express appreciation. Too often we fail to value the importance of communication and end up with communication breakdowns.

Respect healthy, open, and honest communication, and give it the attention it deserves at every level. This means listening, observing, talking, providing feedback, and taking actions that deliver on your words. Quite simply, walk the talk. Never say something you don't mean and don't make promises you aren't willing to keep. Let people know what you expect from them and communicate appreciation for their contributions.

Accountability

People want to be held accountable for their actions. Accountability is part of the structure that helps staff understand you have expectations, will be fair, and will provide a consequence for poor behavior. When bias does not exist and you are respectful, acknowledge accomplishments, and remain consistent in providing constructive criticism and taking punitive actions, you will be respected. Your employees will strive to meet your expectations.

Motivation

Throughout this book, enough has been said about motivating employees. I simply want to stress that it is your responsibility. This is management's point of accountability. If employees aren't motivated, members of the leadership team must look in the mirror, be self-critical, and develop their own performance improvement plan.

TAKE BACK TIME

- *Believe in employees and be there for them.*
- *Learn more about how your employees think in order to inspire top performance.*
- *Explore creative ways to strengthen staff skills, and promote teamwork and longevity.*
- *Respect staff conflict and its invasion on staff's time.*
- *Recognize how to resolve conflicts when they first emerge.*
- *It's the power of CAM—communication, accountability, and motivation—that makes the most of staff's contribution and their time.*

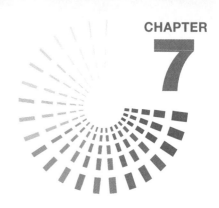
Virtually Yours

*"I think there is a world market
for maybe five computers."*

—*Thomas Watson, IBM Chairman, 1943*

get more excited about technology every day and I am by no means a "techie." I was terrified of my first computer. It was this foreign object over which I had no control, but I stuck with it, because my brain told me it was going to save me lots of time. My brain was right. Of course, like most people I immediately discovered other things to take up that time. Just the same, before I knew it my efficiency doubled. I started working smarter instead of harder.

I have learned to embrace technology. In fact, I eagerly await the arrival of the next great gadget that helps streamline work and provides consistent, reliable outcomes. By the time this book hits the press there will be far more tech tools to help you in the quest to accomplish more with less.

Virtual technology—information technology that works behind the scenes, such as an appointment reminder system—can and should be your new best friend, whether you work in a hospital, ambulatory center, academic practice, large group practice, small group practice, or as a solo practitioner. Information technology, IT, offers unlimited potential to cut costs and improve outcomes with even the most basic tasks. It's the way to achieve reliable and predictable outcomes, manage quality and resources, and improve profitability.

Healthcare leaders must seize every opportunity to improve practice performance, adapt new technologies, and encourage their workers to take advantage of automation. It's all about optimal productivity and giving people the tools to do their jobs better. And it enables you to make the best use of resources without compromising quality.

ANYWHERE, ANYTIME

Not so long ago, accessing information that resided within the practice—whether it was from the practice management system or from the electronic medical record—meant talking to someone who was in the office or going to the office yourself. With virtual technology, you can examine those records from any location, as long as you have access to a computer and Internet access.

Get plugged in by going online and using the office's computer system when you are not in the office. A perfect example is www.gotomypc.com, which enables you to access your computer from home or elsewhere at your convenience. Think about this. It's not just you; you can actually have some staff members work off-site, making work more convenient for them and eliminating interruptions that reduce productivity when employees are on-site. Depending upon your culture and the adaptation to technology in the practice, this could be a great option.

SMART SOURCING

Smart sourcing means being strategic and smart about what you outsource, so time is gained and money is saved. There are two primary ways to gain time and "smart source" by virtually offloading work. The first is implementing technology that can be managed on- or off-site. The second is to simply outsource the entire process.

TAKE IT TO THE BANK

Here are some smart sourcing, smart-thinking suggestions you can take to the bank. Table 1 presents a few examples of how you can use technology to save time. Certainly you can apply virtual technology to many more functions in order to streamline the workload throughout the office.

In the few tasks outlined in Table 1 you can see that there are 60% fewer processes with automation, which saves valuable time, reduces the chance for errors, and expedites the outcome.

Think about the rote tasks and manual processes that eat away at staff time, and explore which technologies can reduce administrative burdens.

How about the amount of work involved for your billing staff to manually track outstanding claims and send tracers, or in the case of patient balances, follow up on delinquent accounts? Your existing practice management system may be able to do this, or it may be more cost-effective to outsource it. It's certainly worth the time to investigate your options and their potential return on investment. When these processes are automated you are bound to improve cash flow and better manage the revenue cycle.

When it comes to controlling costs and saving time, online shopping is a great tool. Everything from office supplies to clinical supplies and equipment can be priced and purchased online at your convenience. Medical practice leaders tell me they have experienced an impressive cut in medical supply costs with online services at www.esurg.com. Online shopping reduces the time otherwise spent meeting with vendors or playing telephone tag.

Let Me Count the Ways

Technology ideas for your office are plentiful. An esteemed colleague of mine, Rosemarie Nelson, MS, an information technology specialist and consultant

TABLE 1. Comparison of Technology Processes

Function	Manual System: Low Tech	Automation: High Tech
Payroll	1. Gather time cards 2. Calculate hours worked and accumulated paid time off 3. Calculate deductions 4. Prepare and distribute payroll checks 5. Prepare and distribute estimated taxes 6. Manage recordkeeping	1. Upload records from time clock electronically 2. Computerize tracking of data 3. Automatically deposit employee and tax payments
Claims Payments	1. Distribute and open mail 2. Post payments and adjustments 3. Endorse checks 4. Prepare deposits 5. Take deposits to bank 6. File explanations of benefits (EOBs) and other supporting documentation	1. Automatically forward mail-in patient payments directly to bank lock box, and third party payments through bank lock box or electronic claims remittance (ECR) 2. Make bank deposits and provide verification, e-copies of checks, EOBs and other documents 3. Post payments and adjustments
Patient Statements	1. Print statements 2. Add dunning messages 3. Fold statements and stuff envelopes 4. Affix postage 5. Mail	1. Upload statements to third party service
Check Preparation	1. Examine and verify invoices and statements 2. Prepare checks 3. Obtain authorized signatures 4. Prepare envelope 5. Fold checks and stuff envelopes 6. Affix postage 7. Mail 8. File documents	1. Examine and verify invoices and statements 2. Submit payments online 3. Scan documents
Insurance Verification and Referrals	1. Check manual for phone and contact person 2. Place phone call 3. Spend undetermined wait time on hold 4. Verify benefits verbally 5. Write down pertinent data	1. Go online to company 2. Verify needed data 3. Print copy

for the Medical Group Management Association gives a number of examples in her presentation "40 Tech Ideas in 40 Minutes," delivered at Pri-Med conferences across the country in 2007. Everything from the personal data assistant (PDA) to the slick all-in-one device centers that integrate a fax, copier, scanner, and printer for the nurse stations are readily available and practical for the medical office. With the ability to move data between insurance carriers and the practice, and between practices and hospitals or diagnostic centers, the benefits of using new technologies just get better. The virtual world continually aids the healthcare industry with quantum leaps that enable practices to make better use of their time, and that provide tools that help you serve and care for the patients.

VIRTUAL I.Q.

Most consumers are accustomed to using virtual technology, accomplishing a variety of tasks through commands that enable one computer to talk to another. They make airline reservations, check the weather, follow their investments, and gather medical information on the Internet. Technology is now part of our everyday life, and we are far more comfortable with virtual activities than a few years back. It's the perfect time to add more technology to healthcare for interactions with patients. Don't hang on to the old way of doing things because "that's the way we've always done it" or "our patients like it this way." It's time to make better use of technology in the office. It's time to shift into high gear with virtual, computer-based applications.

Virtually Speaking

Look at cell phones—even Granny has one. We use cell phones to talk, leave voice mail messages, go online, text message and send photos that we shoot with the cell phone's camera. More savvy business folks combine other technology to their cell phone, including e-mail, appointment schedules, and reminders. So, let's look at ways you can use virtual technology to better communicate with your patients.

Start with improving the way you manage appointments. Recently I suggested to one of my clients that the practice move to an automated reminder system, only to hear the response, "Our patients would never go for this. They want to hear from one of our staff." This may have been true in the past, but the virtual I.Q. of your patients has advanced at an amazing rate over the past ten years. They want information fast and at their convenience, and they want it electronically. E-communication has arrived, is here to stay, and has gained sophisticated capabilities in recent years.

An automated telephone reminder system cuts the workload for staff and improves efficiency. You can reach patients in the way that they prefer to be reached: at work, home, by cell phone, voice mail or text messaging, or via e-mail. It's consistent and reliable.

An effective telephone reminder system eliminates hours of staff time and reduces the no-show rate, which costs the average practice thousands of dollars each month. Cellminder, (www.cellminder.com) is revolutionizing the sophistication and flexibility of one-way communication from practice to patient with virtual communication solutions that help manage cancellations, fill gaps in the schedule, and send customized messages to provide patients with instructions or other information. The tracking tools and customized reports make it easier and more consistent for you to monitor appointment activities and patient compliance with medical treatment.

I'll be covering a lot more about technology and your patients in chapter 8, "Your Ultimate Partner: The Patient," in which the use of a patient portal with interactive features will be discussed. These features promise to improve communication, patient satisfaction, and staff productivity while saving time, improving communication, and moving information faster.

Virtual technology can enhance communication within the office as well. If you aren't using instant messaging and e-mail, you are missing the boat. Virtual communication between staff and physicians will save everyone steps. It will keep staff working at their desk rather than wandering the halls to talk to someone or get answers to their questions.

What about playing a message when patients are on hold? It beats subjecting them to music that may not be of their preference. You can choose the information you want the patients to hear. On-hold messaging is an inexpensive and efficient way to provide general information to your patients. Check out www.intellisound.net.

On-hold messaging enhances communication between the office and the patient. If you treat the senior population, why not remind patients to get their flu shots in the fall? In an obstetrics-gynecology practice, consider a message to remind women of the importance of getting a mammogram at a specific age, or to recommend that prenatal care begin in the first trimester. Dermatologists favor reminding their patients to use sunscreen and letting callers know about newly available cosmetic procedures. Look for a message-on-hold service that is accustomed to working with medical practices and can provide the flexibility needed to customize and change messages with ease.

You can also reduce the number of inbound phone calls for patients inquiring about their lab results. Lab Calls at www.labcalls.com gives patients the opportunity to call in and obtain the results to their tests based on your approval. Of course, not every patient will want to do this; but remember that as time moves on, patients are becoming accustomed to using automated systems to obtain information. They can retrieve the results at their convenience, eliminating the frustration of playing telephone tag.

EMR AND MORE

There are partial electronic solutions a practice can implement before they are ready to fully adopt an electronic medical record, EMR. E-prescribing alone reduces those many steps required in a manual system to take the message, retrieve the chart (which may not be filed), send the chart to the provider, make the call or fax the prescription to the pharmacy, document in the chart, route the chart to medical records, and file the chart. E-prescribing also expedites the outcome, ending those repeat calls from either the pharmacy or the patient.

EMR, also referred to as electronic health records (EHR), certainly requires a greater financial investment. But having access to data; reducing costs involved with transcription, storing, and retrieving charts and records management; and improving practice productivity are enticing incentives.

With EMR physicians learn to document patient care as it is given. This allows physicians and other healthcare providers to move swiftly through the day, staying on time and getting out of the office on time!

The EMR allows physicians to access medical records virtually with a tablet computer or a PDA, improving their ability to respond to a patient's medical needs without delay. Physicians can even complete their hospital charge reporting in real time. This ensures charges are not dropped and are reported both accurately and rapidly—providing a boost to the practice's cash flow.

Just the Facts

Physicians are looking to EMR for convenience and efficiency. *The Electronic Health Records Trends and Usage Survey,* conducted by the Medical Records Institute in 2006, reveals some interesting facts regarding the driving force for medical practices making the EMR decision.

• Of those who responded to the survey, 81.7% were seeking efficiency and

TABLE 2. Adoption of Electronic Health Records

Group Size	Percent with EMR
Five or fewer full-time equivalent (FTE) physicians	12.5%
Six to ten FTE physicians	15.2%
11 to 19 FTE physicians	18.9%
20 or more FTE physicians	19.5%

Source: Data from MGMA study of 3,300 medical group practices, Assessing Adoption of Health Information Technology.

convenience through remote access, which enhanced work flow benefits by reducing interruptions from the pharmacy and patients about refills, lab results, etc.

● A majority—60%—of the respondents wanted to save and increase revenue through better coding and charge capture, as well as decreased manual transcription.

● Over half (52.6%) wanted to gain the satisfaction of patients and physicians.

● Respondents were aware of the need for change, with 44.4% recognizing that they need to survive and thrive in a much more competitive, interconnected world.

This is very revealing and strongly implies that medical practices understand that it is a smart business decision to invest in EMR.

Studies vary on the number of physicians that are adopting EMRs. A study conducted by MGMA[1] indicates that 14.1% of all group practices are using EMR systems. The larger practices are further along in this migration than their peers, as indicated in Table 2.

Many medical practices that have been reluctant to implement EMR systems in the past are either exploring their options or taking the plunge now. According to a study[2] conducted several years ago, 25% of office-based physicians reported that they are using or are in the process of adopting EMR systems. Another 34% of the respondents reported that they plan to implement electronic medical records within two years. So it's fair to assume that more than 60% of medical practices nationwide will have EMR in place in a few short years.

---

[1] *Assessing Adoption of Health Information Technology*, MGMA, September 2005.
[2] Centers for Disease Control and Prevention/National Center for Healthcare Statistics, National Ambulatory Medical Care Study, 2005.

EMR is expected to be an essential component of future pay for performance (P4P) programs adopted by government, major insurance payers, and large employers. The Center for Medicare Services (CMS) P4P pilot programs include an incentive for adoption of the electronic medical record.

EMR provides business intelligence not otherwise available. It facilitates the gathering of accurate clinical data to examine clinical performance and analyze clinical outcomes across the continuum of care.

Getting Started

If you are committed to implementing an EMR system, assign a project team. It is best to have a clinician head the team. To gain a clear picture of the benefits the practice hopes to gain with EMR, the project team will need to gather information about the staff, patients, and how work flows in your existing paper world.

Know what you don't know.

Gather baseline data about how the current paper chart is being used. Are the people that now access the records the ones who will be doing so when you go electronic? This is the time to identify the processes that are riddled with error, redundancy, and inefficiencies, and address those problems before you migrate to a paperless record. Transitioning to EMR is reengineering the processes, and there has to be a bridge between what you are doing now and what you will do in the future.

In addition to charting and accommodating charge entry, there's no doubt that EMR will make a number of daily tasks easier by managing phone calls and prescriptions, and through the ease with which the on-call physician can access the patient's records. Just the same, it requires changes in the way the practice currently does business.

Change is never easy. It requires careful planning. For this you need a champion—someone in the organization who will be the EMR advocate and bring people along when progress stalls. Involve staff. If they will be affected by the decision, they need to be aware of what is going to happen and they need to be heard. Their buy-in is critical to a successful integration.

Learn from Others

Before you take the leap, talk to the practices that have gone before you. Their experience with implementing EMR solutions will help you avoid mistakes and direct you toward reliable vendors. It's important to seek vendors with a product that meets your needs and a dependable customer service performance record.

It is easy to struggle with how to get started when there are so many EMR vendors reaching out to get your business. The advice and experience of other practices will help you better define your needs and narrow the possible vendor list. It is best to limit your in-depth analysis to four to five systems, selecting companies that have been providing EMR solutions to medical practices for at least five years. Determine what additional criteria are important to the practice in selecting these four or five systems you want to consider, and explore further. For example, some practices think it's important to have a vendor that is in their geographic area, while others simply want to make sure customer service is available during the hours they are typically open, regardless of where the vendor's corporate office is located. On the other hand, you may feel it is vital to select a company that has a large customer base in your specialty. If you have a limited budget, price may be the important issue, and with that in mind you are willing to forgo all the bells and whistles more sophisticated systems have to offer.

Once you've interviewed the vendors, completed the demos, and received written proposals, there's still more homework to be done. Turn to reliable sources for help and information before you make a final selection. With a little online research you will discover a number of tools to help you through the decision-making process. Physicians Practice, www.physicianspractice.com, is a great resource for gathering information. The Health Information and Management Systems Society offers an EMR selection tool that is available at www.ehrselector.com.

In my experience, when a practice is disenchanted with its EMR system, it is not because of the software itself, but is more likely due to one or more of the following reasons:

- Lack of commitment from all physicians.
- Poor planning and implementation.
- Unsatisfactory vendor support and customer service.

EMR is a major capital investment, so you may want to consider working with a healthcare consultant who has IT experience. Not only can the consultant guide you through the selection process, she will play an important role in preparing you for and leading you through the implementation process and adjusting to the changes involved.

ABOVE AND BEYOND

I think one of our greatest concerns with technology relates to how fast it is advancing. We recognize that new advancements are always just around the corner and fear that an investment in new technology will be antiquated before its time. This can result in putting off a decision to integrate new technology into the office, whether it's a upgrading the practice management system, adding an EMR solution, or purchasing a new laser or ultrasound. If we wait, it is likely that:

- The technology will become more sophisticated.
- We will get more for our money.
- The costs will come down.
- What we bought will quickly become obsolete.

These reasons to postpone purchasing new technology seem valid, but in reality waiting means we are willing to live with our inefficient manual systems, the burden these systems place on everyone, and the ways that manual systems compromise our time. Remember—time is money!

What Does the Future Hold?

Technology promises to bring more tools to the healthcare industry. These tools designed to improve work efficiency, patient care, and customer service, while containing the cost of healthcare. With the application of technology, a more robust medical practice emerges.

The best way to prepare for the future and know what's on the horizon is to stay connected. Network with peers and attend conferences that provide information on emerging technologies and the projected implications for enhancing medical practice performance.

Beyond this, continue to take a critical look at practice performance to identify areas in which efficient workflow is compromised. Ask that old question, "Is there a better mousetrap?" Seek to find that better solution, and turn to the experts who understand medical practice needs and stay abreast of technological advancements—someone who has been successful in implementing technology solutions.

The Holy Grail

According to Rosemarie Nelson, a principal consultant with MGMA, "The holy grail is the integrated EHR, which supports interoperability within the care community. It aggregates the total care experience electronically."[3] The integrated EHR eliminates the fragmentation that now exists with patient health records and the inability for physicians to access medical records across the continuum of care when making medical decisions. It's in our future, it's attainable!

THE LAST WORD

Virtual technology and smart sourcing offer excellent opportunities to keep your staff performing well, while the practice refines processes and stream-lines costs. Technology provides a means to improve results and provide better service to the patients. It stands to reason that IT solutions will continue to support and advance business and clinical performance in the healthcare industry. Cutting-edge technology products emerge every day. It's our responsibility to keep an open mind and be enthusiastic about the opportunities technology continues to offer.

Sure, tech tools cost money, but the return on investment can sometimes be huge. One thing is sure: if you fail to keep up with technology, the competition will pass you by and the cost of doing business will continue to rise. There's no slow lane on the information highway, so buckle your seat belt and enjoy the ride. ●

TAKE BACK TIME

- *Technology improves precision with business and clinical performance.*
- *Virtual technology moves information accurately and swiftly, saving time and money.*
- *Don't let manual systems bog you down.*
- *Smart-source by adding virtual technology and outsourcing.*
- *Technology reduces processes and increases efficiency.*
- *Careful planning is essential to EMR migration.*
- *The holy grail is an integrated EMR system across the continuum of care.*
- *Be enthusiastic about emerging technologies that improve business and clinical performance.*

---

[3] Rosemarie Nelson, "Tech Tips," *MGMA Directions*, Spring 2006, 6(4):4.

Your Ultimate Partner—
The Patient

*"Alone we can do so little;
together we can do so much."*

—*Helen Keller*

The idea of partnering with your patients is a concept that takes on different meanings for each of us. Some physicians may fear it gives patients more control or too much power in the clinical arena. Some haven't a clue on the theory behind the concept of developing "partnering" avenues and how this would benefit both patients and the practice. Then again, there are those physicians that simply have the knack—they know just how to go about developing and nurturing the patient relationship and turning it into a true partnership.

How physicians practice medicine is not my business. But I am in the business of helping medical practices, surgery and diagnostic centers, hospitals, and health systems use the resources they have to do the best they can for the patients, the staff, and themselves. Partnering with the patients helps accomplish this and effectively saves time. It's an excellent way to ensure you are both on the same team, work collectively for the benefit of the patient's health, and avoid barriers.

Some barriers are outside the realm of what happens within the medical setting. They are affected by politicians, advocacy groups, corporations, and America's overriding concerns about rising healthcare costs. Other barriers are processes within the practice that are influenced by the actions of professionals whose mission is to serve the patients.

UNDERSTAND YOUR PATIENTS

The better physicians and the healthcare team understand their patients—the way they think, what drives their concerns or actions, and what they want from you—the better you will be able to help them, and the better they will be able to deal with their healthcare issues.

The dynamics of the patients' attitudes and their impressions and respect toward the medical community is fluid. It is ever-changing, for obvious reasons. It depends on the patient experience—everything from the first impression to the last encounter with you or the people that represent you. Through our own actions, we have the ability to influence the patient's attitude and strengthen the relationship.

Early Beginnings

Patients and their caregivers often form their opinions early on. It starts with the way you communicate and set their expectations. Take Superb Hospital's

ad campaign and the print copy advertising placed in the local paper. It may
be a fabulous ad, giving the reader the impression that Superb is as com-
forting and warm as a childhood teddy bear. Now, what if Mrs. Pleasant's experience includes an indifferent staff, cold food that is not what she ordered,
a medication error, and a failure to meet even her smallest request? So much
for warm and fuzzy care. I've seen this happen—and it was happening in a
hospital that bragged about its VIP service!

Then there's First Class Medical Practice. They have a slick brochure
and a fabulous Website that almost guarantees a first-class experience for
the patient. Besides this, the senior physician has been interviewed in
the local media many times and is considered a guru in his specialty.
Now what if Mr. Concerned arrives and finds the office aesthetics dis-
mal, out of date, and poorly maintained? The receptionists are wearing
scrubs that look like slept-in pajamas, Mr. Concerned is greeted by a
sign-in sheet, and no one calls him by name. In addition, he waits forty
minutes, the office failed to tell him he was scheduled with the junior partner, and he gets rushed through the visit. This surely doesn't feel like
the first class service he imagined.

In both these scenarios the patient's expectations were set in advance and
were not met. If your practice's attitude, physical presence, and actions don't
live up to the image you initially portrayed, barriers to building an effective
partnership begin to emerge. The patient may feel betrayed, or at the very
least, disappointed. His attitude shifts as he experiences negative feelings.

- Agitation
- Mistrust
- Impatience

This can result in an uncooperative or demanding patient. Addressing
his disappointment will take up valuable time that could otherwise be dedicated to developing a mutually beneficial relationship.

Be careful what you promise or imply. Developing a good relationship
starts with matching expectations, making the patient feel valued, and delivering a satisfactory experience and outcome. The image you portray should
match your mission and core values. A mission is not just a lofty statement,
it is the very purpose of your organization and it's vitally important to take
concrete steps to live the mission.

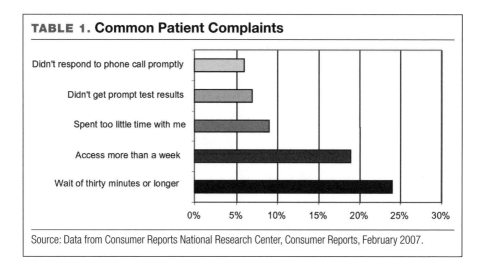

TABLE 1. Common Patient Complaints

Source: Data from Consumer Reports National Research Center, Consumer Reports, February 2007.

WHAT BUGS PATIENTS

In a recent study conducted by *Consumer Reports*, patients spoke up about what bothers them about their physicians; see Table 1. The results are revealing. Each one of these indicators relates to time—you are not respecting theirs.

The Truth

Patients want you to care, and they want the truth. That may seem bewildering to some of my readers. After all, I'm sure you care about the patients and you certainly don't lie to them. The truth is in your actions, and it doesn't always match what you say or attempt to portray. When your words and actions don't match, patients become disenchanted and may even feel a sense of betrayal.

Take Action Now

Start by taking the five indicators in Table 1. Now change hats. If you were a patient going somewhere for care, how long would you be willing to wait without being annoyed? Set tentative time-frame standards for each indicator.

Next, track your own performance. It's fairly simple. Count the incidences of each indicator for five days and find out how often you actually hit the benchmark—your stated goal or acceptable standard. In other words, what's the ratio? If you saw 100 patients but failed to meet the standard/goal thirty times, the goal was only reached 70% of the time. Set your expectation high, at least 90%. If you don't hit the mark, do something about it.

Establish intervention strategies to improve outcomes in the areas where your performance is sub-par.

Tell It Like It Is

When it comes to communication with patients, for heaven's sake, let the patient know what to expect. When a patient will need to wait for a telephone response, it's your employee's responsibility to tell him how long the wait will be. "Mr. Concerned, Dr. Care returns her calls between 11:30 and noon. Will that work for you, and what number do you want her to call?" And how about the anxious patient whose tests you ordered to rule out a potentially severe condition? "Mr. Fearful, we should have the results in seventy-two hours." If you expect the result in forty-eight hours, setting the expectation at seventy-two hours gives you some lead time. It also prevents the patient from calling you before you have the information he wants.

Improving Patient Visit Time

With the help of leadership, physicians around the country are discovering ways to make the most of the patient's visit, in order to improve the patient visit experience and enhance the partnership. This can actually be accomplished in a way that also heightens patient satisfaction and saves time in the long run.

Appointment Scheduling

If access to care takes more than a week, you may need to slot a set number of same-day appointments. A thirty-minute wait to be seen in the office is unreasonable. If patients experience this in your practice or other healthcare setting, it's an efficiency issue or unrealistic scheduling patterns that lead to patients feeling rushed. Either way there are reasonable solutions—so do something about it. It will be more efficient for you and is essential to effectively partnering with your patients.

Visit Preparedness

Medical practices can help patients be more prepared for their visits by giving the patient a list of things to do in advance. Here is a list of common things a patient can do to be ready when they arrive in the office.
1. New patients
   a. Complete medical history forms at home.
   b. Bring copy of the medical record from previous physician.

2. Create a medications list of current medications and dosages.
3. Prepare a list of primary health issues.
4. Develop a list of questions.
5. When the patient needs assistance or a personal advocate, bring along a family member or friend.

So how do you go about this? You can post the visit preparedness tips on your Website, e-mail the list to patients prior to their appointments, or have visit tip sheets available in your reception room. Some practices have a "fill in the blanks" form that patients complete when they are waiting in the reception room.

Shared Decision Making

The term "shared decision making" (SDM), refers to the process of interacting with patients who seek to be more involved in making decisions about testing, screening, and treatment. This is based on the rationale that there is not one clearly indicated best treatment option. SDM aids have emerged as vital tools to strengthen the trust between physicians and patients, improve communication, and encourage the ultimate partnership. The goal of shared decision making is to *give the right care to the right patient at the right time.*

Dartmouth-Hitchcock Medical Center in Lebanon, New Hampshire, championed the SDM concept when it developed the Center for Shared Decision Making. At the center, doctors and decision-making coaches learned to use various decision-making aids to help patients weigh their options. Patients can go online to view Dartmouth's decision aid library and explore materials concerning a variety of conditions.

The article "Shared Decision Making: Benefits and Technology," in the June 2007 issue of *Informed Care Spotlight*, states that shared decision making is gaining significant market adoption, driven by an approach to healthcare that places patients at the center of the continuum. Whether you incorporate SDM into your practice—and the conditions under which SDM may be appropriate—is a professional decision that only you can make.

Anatomy of a Patient

When patients plan to seek medical treatment, their concerns usually relate to fear, time, or money. A hypothetical patient's internal dialogue appears in Table 2.

TABLE 2. Anatomy of a Patient

Fear	• What is really wrong with me? • What if it's serious? • Are the other patients in here contagious? • If I have to be admitted, who will watch the children? • Will it hurt?
Time	• If the doctor doesn't see me soon, I won't be able to pick up the kids when school lets out. • If I miss work, my job will be in jeopardy. • How long will it be before I know what's really wrong? • How much time will I spend running to get tests?
Money	• I can't afford to be sick. • What will this cost me? • I can't afford expensive medications. • How much of this will be covered by insurance? • If I'm off work, there won't be a paycheck.

Think about these concerns and how disturbing it would be to be kept waiting in the reception room, where these concerns seem to become more magnified. This will help you understand the patient's frame of mind and how vulnerable they feel. All of these issues can become bigger than life for patients who are kept waiting, who think you are indifferent, who feel that communication with them is poor, or who feel their time is not valued by the practice staff—the people they now depend upon for their health. The message here is to treat the patient, not just the condition.

BE PATIENT-FRIENDLY

It's not your job to be friends with the patients, but it is your responsibility to be friendly to them. Treat patients as you would a guest in your home. Greet them, make sure they are comfortable, and be kind and attentive.

Healthcare leaders and physicians set the tone for staff. Employees will mimic the behavior of their leaders. If you treat both the employees and the patients respectfully and you honor their time, the employees will want to treat the patient this way.

On the other hand, if you fail to say good morning to staff, force them to put their personal life on hold to work overtime, exhibit a poor attitude and say unkind things, or if you fail to listen to their needs, this lack of respect will transfer to similar negative actions toward the patients.

The Mantra

Each person interacting with the patient can demonstrate a patient-friendly commitment simply by asking the patient at the end of the encounter, "Is there anything else I can do for you today?" We tend to think this will slow us down, but in reality it just keeps us working in real-time and limiting the potential for unanswered questions that result in a disruptive phone call or additional actions later on.

Patient Satisfaction

If you don't ask, you don't know how satisfied your patients are. Sure there are some indicators, like patients who refer their friends, those who always seem pleased, and those who give positive feedback to their referring physicians. But these are mere observations of a small sampling of your patient base. Your impressions just might be off the mark.

It is important to measure patient satisfaction in a way that ensures the data is not skewed and the results not compromised. If patients complete surveys at the time of their visits, the same person may repeatedly respond to the survey. This also limits the sampling to voluntary participation, making it unclear whether the sampling is representative of the practice's patient population. The survey results become biased, unreliable, and useless.

Some experts suggest that patient satisfaction surveys be conducted and analyzed by a professional surveyor who is unrelated to your organization. This requires an investment, but it is essential to obtaining and analyzing reliable quantitative information. Once you have acquired baseline results, you can set specific improvement goals to help the practice reach higher levels of patient satisfaction.

The Sounding Board

Unhappy patients need somewhere to go with their complaints; otherwise their complaints become "gripes" that everyone hears but no one addresses, creating a negative environment and lowering productivity, morale, and patient satisfaction. You can avert this problem by providing a sounding board for your patients—a dispute resolution process.

By implementing a method for patients to register complaints in private, where they are heard and solutions are offered, patients will feel you really care. A dispute resolution system also provides an opportunity to obtain qualitative information about patients' complaints, so you will know where you stand with customer service.

An incident report needs to be completed for each dispute. The report should describe the complaint and the measures taken to resolve it. Keep a control copy on file, and you'll be able to periodically analyze the issues that emerged over time, who was involved, the seriousness of the problem, what corrective actions were taken, and the time-frame required to reach resolution. By reviewing trends over time, you'll be able to develop an internal report card. It's an important tool for examining the practice's commitment to resolving patient disputes and maintaining a patient-friendly culture.

SUPPORTING EACH OTHER

The best-run organizations have a team culture. The team consists of physicians and other healthcare providers, management, staff, and the patients. Each person has an important role, and they support each other to get things done—efficiently, in a timely manner, and with a quality outcome. It's all about supporting one another and looking for opportunities to work toward the common good of the team.

Advocates

Advocacy is important in terms of guiding results to help achieve the desired outcome, while protecting the interest of others. Advocates work in partnership with others; to make the ultimate partnership, a practice can formally assign someone in the practice to be the patient advocate.

The patient advocate is the person that looks out for the patient's interest, takes note when the patient-friendly service begins to decline, and brings problems to leadership's attention.

The patient advocate is the "go to" person for patients. When a patient has a special request, the advocate will help find the most appropriate solution. Sometimes it involves an outside entity. For example, a patient may have trouble understanding the multiple bills they receive from different sources following a hospitalization. The advocate will either answer the questions and clear the matter up or lead the patient to someone that can.

The patient advocate is a great resource to help identify when there are other products or services you might want to offer the patients, such as in-house testing, nutritional supplements, or ancillary services.

Your Best Ally

When the patient is a practice advocate, she becomes an extension of you in the community. This is often exhibited informally when current patients refer new patients to you. A patient that endorses you to friends, family, and co-workers and recommends they seek care from you is your advocate and best ally.

The patient can become a great advocate in other situations as well. For example, if you are having problems getting paid by a particular third party plan, consider asking the patient to get involved. She can contact the customer service department and seek a remedy, or in the case of an employer sponsored health plan, the patient can go directly to the employer and register her concern.

Practices are offloading tasks that patients are willing and able to handle, such as obtaining x-rays or medical records from other providers prior to their appointment, or scheduling off-site ancillary studies. This saves the practice time, and patients don't have to wait for you to get around to it. They are also able to schedule the appointment at their convenience and get firsthand instructions. It reduces steps and the potential for miscommunications that sometimes result in errors. Of course it's important for you to have an internal mechanism in place to monitor patient compliance. For example, if you order a study on a patient and you'd like him to get it within the week, why not schedule a two-week follow up appointment and ask the patient to bring a copy of the results with him? If you have an electronic reminder system on the computer, you can enter the patient's study on the reminder system so they either get a phone call, you call the patient to make sure they've completed the study, or you check the chart to see if the report is in the file. There are other methods to stay on top of this, but the more automated the better.

TECHNOLOGY AND YOUR PATIENT

Many of you have already noticed that savvy patients are surfing the Internet. They are getting information about the hospitals and physicians in their community; they are getting information about services and medical conditions;

and they are making decisions based on the information they obtain. It's happening behind the scenes and it's powerful.

This section will provide stimulating ways for you to communicate and enrich the patient relationship through technology. It starts with asking patients for their e-mail address as a way to keep in touch—to communicate and serve them better. Update the patient registration form to include asking for the patient's e mail addresses. That takes care of the new patients, but you'll also need to obtain e-mail addresses from your established patients when they call in or have a visit.

Medical practices have been slow to recognize the advantages of implementing e-communication with their patients. E-mail is a great way for the patient advocate to receive and provide information to the patient and to expedite resolution. E-mail saves time and improves service, but as with most things it requires proper planning and a commitment.

The reception room kiosk is emerging as a check-in tool for patients when they arrive at the medical practice. Galvanon's system (www.galvanon. com) allows the patient to check in and verify demographics, such as updating their address, phone, employment, and insurance information. Depending on the level of sophistication of the kiosk, patients may be able to not only view their appointment on the computer's monitor and check themselves in but also make their co-payment, much like we are accustomed to doing with airlines.

Make It Easy

The application of the technology must be user-friendly and uncomplicated to permit the patients to use it with ease. There will still be a learning curve for staff and patients which may require more time or resources during the transition.

You will need to do some hand-holding, based on how much technology your patients have adapted to in their daily lives. Administratively, many patients check on their insurance benefits and participating physicians online. They even explore the Websites of the providers before making their choices.

Patients have been keeping records of their own healthcare for a long time. Parents carry a notebook with the toddler's immunizations and a diary of illnesses and medications. Patients with chronic illnesses are accustomed to monitoring medications, flares, and complications and hospitalizations. Hypertensive patients monitor their blood pressure and heart rate, diabetics keep a constant eye on glucose levels, and asthmatic patients know how to manage their condition. They are ready to use technology more and they want more information about their health. Patients are accustomed to coordinating their own healthcare between providers and transferring information. They are ready for a patient health record, PHR. Are you?

THE WEBSITE ROADMAP

Your Website should contribute to the ultimate partnership. By providing important information to the patients through your Website, you reduce phone calls while patients get the information they want, when they want it. The Website should be professionally designed, including both the graphics and the written content.

Vital Statistics

Start with simple things like listing your location[s] and office hours, contact information, and brief biographical sketches about the physicians, including training and experience.

You'll want to list the hospitals where the physicians have staff privileges and the insurance plans with which you contract. This also gives you an opportunity to define your basic patient financial policy.

Other important items to include on the Website are your mission statement and core values.

Communicate

A top-notch Website becomes a valuable communication tool. Its flexibility and the versatility depends on the depth of information you want to provide.

Some practices add a question-and-answer section to the Website to address patients' most common concerns, based on specialty and the types of conditions the practice typically treats. You may want to provide seasonal reminders for groups of people, such as advising patients to get their flu shot in the fall, or the dermatologist might want to suggest the annual mole check in the spring. Your website can also lead patients (through links) to reliable sources of clinical information about their medical conditions. If you don't provide the link, they will get information elsewhere on the Internet, possibly from sources that are not reliable or simply unknown.

Patient Portals

Patient portals are virtual doors into your practice. With the proper firewalls and encryption, they become a practical way to better serve patients while saving you time. Patients can interact with your practice without a phone call, reducing the labor-intensive processes involved with telephone communication.

By accessing the portal (and depending on which services you decide to offer online), patients can request appointments, prescription renewals, and referrals. They can even access test results.

Patients will actually be able to complete patient registration forms and the patient history on their computer and upload them to your office, where the information becomes part of the patient's record. The information can be reviewed and verified when the patient comes into the office. This saves time otherwise dedicated for staff to enter the information on the patient's record by writing on hard copies or typing data into the patient's electronic medical record.

Bring It On

Think about activities in the office that can be automated and bring it on. Seek automated solutions that will reduce the number of steps required, limit the potential for error, and accomplish the desired result more quickly.

Now it's time to move the office and the Website forward by developing a patient technology integration plan. It will include your personal selection of what technology best suits your practice, resources that are needed to implement, steps required, and a projected time frame to complete the transition.

Considerations:
1. Patient registration
2. Appointment scheduling, where you set the criteria
3. Completion of health history forms
4. Account query
5. Payment
6. E-mail

Direct Patients

There are a number of ways you can influence patients to access the Website for information and to use the interactive components.

- Add the Web address to print materials: stationery, appointment cards, patient registration form, consent forms, etc.
- Direct patients to the Website through the inbound telephone script.
- Staff can remind patients to visit the Website.
- Include the Web address on marketing materials.
- Create a three-minute patient video on the home page of the Website. The video can tout the Website features and the advantages it offers the patients.
- Think about creating a video loop for your reception area that points patients to the Website.

Don't Abuse

Don't let technology replace the personal touch or threaten the patient-friendly culture that strives to exceed patients' expectations.

Approach change cautiously and closely monitor the patients' reactions and acceptance of your initiatives. Advance at the patients' pace, not yours—and give them whatever support and reassurance is needed to make the partnership work. ●

TAKE BACK TIME

- *Don't set unrealistic expectations.*
- *Set performance standards that value patients' time.*
- *When it comes to your service culture, leadership sets the tone for staff.*
- *A patient-friendly practice saves time.*
- *Shift some tasks to the patients.*
- *Enhance your Website with features that communicate with and educate your patients.*
- *Implement interactive technology at the patient's pace.*

Mine the Business

"Humans only use ten percent of the brain and seven percent of company databases, yet we're always one hundred percent sure of everything. That just doesn't add up."

— *Christine Bultnick*

ere we are living in an instant society where we want things at our fingertips and available to us at all times. We do this in business as well as in our personal lives. Today we have an enormous advantage over the healthcare leaders and decision makers of twenty years ago. We have access to reliable and accurate data, data that can be captured, used to drive business decisions, and help us protect the interests of the business owners, workers, and customers.

Here's the problem. Because we get distracted with the day-to-day operations and solving the daily crises, we sometimes fail to focus on mining the data and minding the business!

HOW ARE DECISIONS MADE NOW?

How decisions are made seems like a simple question, but it stymies me that when I meet individually with the leaders of a medical group, each person is likely to give me a different answer. I have discovered that with the exception of large medical groups and institutions, many decisions are made in an ad hoc manner based on subjective information and current circumstances. Too often decisions are made in an effort to resolve an existing crisis or to placate an individual or group of people. Crisis management leads to making decisions that are not thought out and that can be harmful, wasting a great deal of time and resources. In reality, many crisis situations can be avoided with better planning and by making data-driven decisions.

Business Intelligence

Business intelligence (BI) refers to a process of making intelligent use of available data in decision making. In order to accomplish this you must extract electronic data from the various systems where it is stored, link the useful facts, and filter out irrelevant data.

Historically, smart businesses have used data to drive decisions. However, before the evolution of computers it was a laborious, manual process riddled with the potential for significant errors. The emergence of "business intelligence" and use of historical data to forecast and make intelligent decisions has become more commonplace with the integration of technology into most facets of business operations. Today you can gather reliable data to better understand your organization's performance and determine what strategic actions would be in your best interest, support your mission, and help the organization achieve its goals. Table 1 explains the components of BI.

TABLE 1. The Components of Business Intelligence	
Situation Awareness	Filtering out irrelevant information and synthesizing the relevant data
Risk Assessment	Weighing current and future risk, assessing costs and benefits, and discovering what plausible actions might be taken and when
Decision Support	Using information wisely, providing warning of important events so preventative steps can be taken
Purpose of Business Intelligence	Helping you analyze and make better business decisions, thus improving sales, profitability, customer satisfaction and/or staff morale

BI changes the way we do business in a meaningful way that guides us. This ultimately leads to better decision making and prudent use of our finances, resources, and time.

THE POWER OF DATA

Data mining refers to analyzing data from different sources and different perspectives, and summarizing it into useful information. The value and power of data are dependent on the data we select and how we use it. Know your business—not intuitively, not subjectively, but based upon real data.

Benchmarks

The best-run practices examine specific performance measures that reveal the "state of the practice," and monitor these measures as a report card on how the practice is doing. This is true for the medical practice, diagnostic center, surgery center, dental practice, optometrist, and other varied healthcare providers.

A good snapshot of the practice's performance should include productivity, income, operating expense, and financial management. Typical benchmarks are exhibited in Table 2.

The performance report card is useful in comparing your current performance against past performance. Both month-to-month and information from the same time last year are good comparisons. In addition, for a number of performance elements, internal information can be benchmarked against external data of other practices with similar characteristics, i.e., size, location, and specialty.

Reliable cost surveys, conducted annually by the Medical Group Management Association (MGMA), www.mgma.com, and the National Society of Certified Healthcare Business Consultants (NSCHBC), www.nschbc.org.

TABLE 2. Benchmarks for Assessing Practice Performance

Benchmark	Data	Variables and Factors for Comparison
Productivity	• Charges • Receipts • Adjustments	• Group • Individual provider • Payer class
Receivable Management	• Accounts receivable • Aged receivables	• Group • Individual provider • Days in A/R • By department • By payer class • Percentages/numbers
Profitability	• Income and expense report (or profit and loss, P&L)	• Income • Operating expenses • Net profit • Top ten expenses • Percentage/numbers
Staffing	• Income and expenses report • Payroll records	• Full time equivalents • Costs: percentages and numbers • Turnover • Overtime
Growth and Service Mix	• CPT codes	• New patient ratios • Group • Individual provider • New service • Top evaluation and management (E&M) services • Top ten procedures
Customer Service	• Patient satisfaction surveys • Patient complaints • Patient transfers	• By group • By provider • By type of patient, i.e. age, sex, insurance type, medical condition

These surveys provide data by specialty. NSCHBC statistical reports provide information similar to a typical profit and loss statement in addition to information on charges, adjustments, accounts receivable, and the number of full time equivalent staff. MGMA's survey provides more comprehensive data to perform sophisticated analyses in many areas of practice performance. This benchmarking can be done with ease when MGMA's interactive CD report is purchased.

MGMA's sample size is somewhat small compared to the large database in NSCHBC's statistical report. NSCHBC's report also shows regional data which can provide a useful comparison, and the NSCHBC statistical report includes a broader range of medical specialties as well.

Additional surveys of various areas of practice performance and statistical data may be available through your specialty association, county medical society, regional business alliance, or other professional management organizations.

Graph It

Administrators and practice managers often tell me they run the month-end reports and give them to the physicians, only to discover the physicians don't look at them. Make the data user-friendly by graphing it. Most practice management systems allow you to export the data into an Excel spreadsheet where, with a few clicks of the mouse, it can be presented in bar graphs, scatter grams, or pie graphs.

Most physicians aren't interested in poring over numbers to determine what is meaningful—it simply takes too much time and does not provide an effective cross reference to relevant data. Graphs are your visual message, being both easy to read and easy to understand.

Let Data Tell the Story

Looking at graphs saves time and instantly reveals historical and emerging trends that will help the leadership team keep a pulse on business performance.

Figure 1 is an example of a real client of mine that experienced a troublesome trend mid-year. The significant dip in receipts and spike in adjustments reveals a problem that needed further investigation in order to identify the source of the problem and to protect the practice from a recurrence.

Drilling down data is very revealing and gives you a deeper understanding of both the business position of the practice and its performance.

Figure 2 provides an example of how you can examine accounts receivable performance to understand payer performance. In this example, PPOs represent the lion's share of the pie. To take a closer look at where the money is, the PPO class is drilled down to show individual payer performance (Figure 3). At a glance, it becomes crystal clear that No Way Insurance is the one PPO most untimely in paying claims.

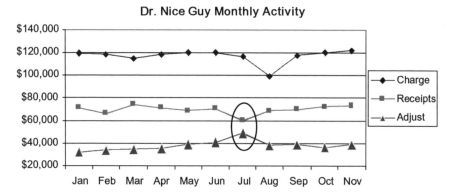

FIGURE 1. Productivity Performance Measures

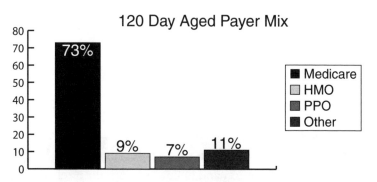

FIGURE 2. Distribution of Aged Accounts Receivable By Payer Class

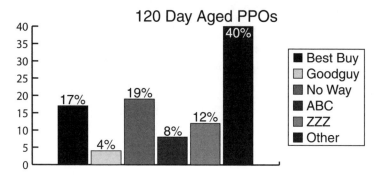

FIGURE 3. Distribution of PPO Aged Accounts Receivable

Dashboards

Dashboards are quickly becoming the "must haves" for savvy business health-care executives, and for good reasons. The dashboard is a metric reporting tool that makes it easy to look at business performance, so you know when the practice is doing well and are alerted when something is wrong. Performance dashboards provide a layered interface that conforms to the way you work. When the dashboard is aligned with the practice's operations, finances, and strategic plan, managers and physicians begin to work more efficiently and effectively toward achieving shared objectives.

Dashboards provide at-a-glance visualization of the company's health and monitoring of key performance indicators. They are simple to understand and easy to use, making them an attractive, popular BI tool.

The BI dashboard is a desktop display similar to the dashboard of your car. It displays important information that you want to monitor. You design it based on the information needs required to keep a pulse on the business. DashboardMD (www.dashboardmd.com)

Dashboard reporting clearly communicates business objectives throughout your organization and allows all users to see the progress toward those goals on a regular basis, which keeps everyone focused and informed. With drilldown capabilities, users may view the desired level of detail, getting the information they need to know and act upon. Dashboards help you monitor the information that you already know is important.

Don't get a dashboard just because it's the latest rage. Make sure you are ready to endorse its function and believe it's something that will reduce the processes currently required to track performance, saving time and elevating your organization's use of data. When developing a customized dashboard, keep it simple and make it relevant!

The MGMA Cost Survey's CD version has a slick dashboard feature that can be implemented in a matter of minutes. It will prepare a dashboard of the practice's performance (per full-time equivalent physician) based on a comparison to your peers around the country with six indicators: revenue, accounts receivable, operating costs, staffing cost, and medical revenue after operating costs. It also provides a percentile ranking to help you understand how your practice measures up.

MAKE SMART DECISIONS

Analyzing critical performance data, properly preparing the information, and using flexible and innovative BI tools will help you with strategic planning, decision-making, and executing strategies to achieve the organization's stated goals. You will stay on target and on time!

Smart Planning and Execution

Mining data is the beginning. The success of executing the data-driven decision requires smart planning—a key component to realistically understanding the capabilities and limitations of the organization, and what resources are required to achieve your goals. This requires a critical examination of strengths, weaknesses, opportunities, and threats—the typical SWOT analysis. Once this is accomplished, develop an action plan that defines what will be done, how results will be measured, who will get the job done, and when you expect it to be completed. This becomes the tool to obtain a commitment, follow progress, and hold people accountable.

Even with the best-laid plans, progress can be thwarted by unexpected events. It's important to monitor progress and know when to shift gears. Otherwise, time and resources can easily be depleted without accomplishing your goals.

Keep Your Eye on the Ball

The business of medicine is moving at lightning speed. It's not enough to just know what's going on inside your business. Keep a pulse on what's happening with competitive factors, consumer attitudes, and political trends that affect your future. Get involved and stay involved. ●

TAKE BACK TIME

- *Crisis management wastes time and resources.*
- *Make intelligent use of data.*
- *Mine data to accomplish an objective analysis.*
- *Graphic presentations of data are powerful.*
- *Let data drive decisions.*
- *Keep dashboards simple and relevant.*

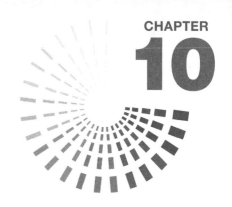

Get Back
Your Life!

*"The purpose of life is
a life of purpose."*

—*Robert Byrne*

This is my favorite chapter of the book. I believe it is the most compelling and could be the right motivation for some of the readers to change bad habits that disrupt or sabotage the potential for a healthy life. We'll see if you agree.

Getting back your life is not a matter of looking at what occupies your time, eliminating some of the time killers, changing a few habits, and going on your merry way. That's a rational approach that seems to make sense, but sooner or later some of us end up right back where we started and wondering how we got there.

To get back your life you must take care of the whole person—body, mind, and spirit.

It's important to nurture and care for each aspect of your life. For many of us, this is not easy to do, but it's achievable and results in a healthier, stronger you.

Are the demands on your time stressful and interfering with the ability to relax, take care of yourself, and find personal fulfillment? If so, it may be an indication that you allow outside influences to control your life and don't have healthy boundaries—boundaries that help keep your personal, family, and professional lives in balance.

If we fail to keep our life in balance, our attitudes change and we become less effective at home and at work. Just think about it. If we fail to accomplish what we set out to do, or if we didn't dedicate time to the areas of our life that create a healthy balance, then frustration and stress mount. A feeling of inadequacy emerges and we are likely to become either defensive or defenseless. Neither of these contributes to us being effective in either our personal or professional lives.

ARE YOU A WORKAHOLIC?

No one starts out as a workaholic. Sometimes it's a result of loving your work, which is not necessarily a bad thing. In fact, loving your work is great. It's where you spend most of your waking hours, and loving work can make you a lot happier when you're not at work. You and I both know that when people aren't happy at work it affects other areas of their life. Loving your work is not the problem—letting work take over your life is.

I remember a discussion I had with an esteemed colleague whom I'll call Amanda. She was telling me about a job she had a few years back, at a place where she worked for more than ten years. She completed her grad-

uate work at a prestigious institution and snagged "the job of a lifetime."
The job provided challenge, responsibility, and opportunity—it also provided long work hours. Amanda was a respected, dedicated employee and
loved her work. In fact, she basked in it, working evenings and weekends
with joy. Before long the only friends she had were the ones at work. She
admitted that in no time at all work became her life, and not without personal and family sacrifices.

After nine years with the company, she began to see signs of trouble at
work. Political issues emerged and talks of restructuring quickly became a
reality. Power plays became evident. Change was constant, and people started
to become insecure and concerned about their future. Not Amanda. Her
job was solid as a rock. Sound familiar? Then it happened—Amanda was
given her walking papers.

Amanda, the workaholic, was devastated and felt she had no purpose.
Her days were empty and the phone wasn't ringing. Her friends went about
with their busy lives with little time to provide much needed comfort.
Amanda had no job and no social life. She also had a luxury she didn't want
and never had before—too much time. The problem is she didn't know
what to do with it. She didn't know how to enjoy the simple things. Her life
had been out of balance for way too long.

Amanda had to learn to take care of herself—body, mind, and spirit,
and take back her life. It was a learning process and a healing process, and
it took a long time to get past the anger and bitterness to seek a healthy,
balanced life.

Many men and women, without realizing it, have let work become their
purpose. They don't even stop to think about how much the job owns them.
I hope you aren't headed in this direction. If so, there's still a way out.

Finding Balance

Give yourself the acid test for a balanced life by understanding how your
life and feeling of self-worth would change if your job vanished in the morning? Would your primary concern about losing the job be the lack of a pay-
check, or would it be a lack of purpose? When your life is in balance, losing
a job is just one element of how you live. It does not define who you are or
your life's purpose. Other than the temporary loss of income, you are able
to get on with your life.

Do what you can to have balance in your life. Life is full of unexpected events. The loss of a job, a need to relocate and leave all that is familiar, a new baby, financial challenges, the empty nest, caring for a frail elderly parent, or a sudden unexpected loss are a few events that might upset the status quo. When faced with a major change, would you be immobilized and have difficulty moving forward? If so, it's time to rebalance your priorities, take care of yourself, and get your life in order.

HEALTHY BOUNDARIES

Last Saturday a friend of mine called while I was working on this book. She said "you must be a workaholic, working on a Saturday." I assured her—and I assure you—that I am not a workaholic. I have healthy boundaries. Most authors will agree that, in order to do their most creative writing, they must be in a creative mood, and when such a mood emerges, they let the creative juices flow. I'm no exception. So on Saturday I worked. The day before I did not work; I had writer's block, so my husband and I went bike riding on the beach. Then this Tuesday I simply took the day off to work on a 1,000-piece puzzle with my granddaughter. I like to play while other people work and frequently I have the luxury of doing that. Life is good!

Having boundaries means knowing when to say yes, when to say no, and learning to take control of your life, according to Dr. Henry Cloud and Dr. John Townsend in their book *Boundaries*.[1] I agree. Yes, you can learn to say no without feeling guilty. Practice! Achieving and maintaining healthy boundaries requires discipline, recognizing what is the right thing to do or right action to take, and knowing when and how to make time for yourself.

When we fail to identify boundaries we end up over-committing. We make promises that are difficult to fulfill, and if fulfilled deplete valuable resources needed elsewhere. Drs. Cloud and Townsend provide a comparison—the *boundary-injured* individuals and the *boundary-developed* individuals. Those that are boundary-injured either resentfully make good on their promises or they fail to deliver, and are left guilt-ridden. Boundary-developed people make good on their promises freely and gladly, or they simply don't promise at all! Makes sense, doesn't it?

---

[1] Cloud H. and Townsend J. *Boundaries.* Zondervan, Grand Rapids, Michigan, 1992.

Time Fit

My favorite definition of the word "fit" in the *New World Dictionary* is "to be in accord or harmony." It's a marvelous description we can apply to balancing time. Being "time fit" is all about using time wisely in all areas of your life—keeping that healthy balance we strive to achieve.

Much of this book has focused on the use of time at work, but to know if we are time fit, we must look at our time off the job. Most of us look forward to the weekend and getting away from work. By the time Friday rolls around we already have plans for the weekend. Our time intentions may involve relaxation, entertainment, home improvement projects, or time with family and friends. Now get up close and personal with what really happens to our time.

Examine your personal time intentions by looking backward and forward. Reflect on last Friday when you had eagerly looked forward to your plans for the weekend. What were those exact plans? How many of those things happened as planned? How many were derailed, and why? This is the acid test for whether you are time fit. Here are some typical reasons we fail to fulfill our personal plans, and these causes could be equally responsible for how time is managed on the job.

- We fail to make the plan a priority.
- We feel guilty.
- We bring work home.
- We are unrealistic about what can be accomplished.
- We didn't allow for predictable interruptions, things that happen routinely over a weekend.
- We have unhealthy boundaries.

What I find alarming is how often we find it perfectly acceptable that we don't get to do what we want with our free time, but too often beat ourselves up when we don't get everything done at work. The road to being time fit might be a long one, but here are a few ideas on how to get started.

Personally Yours

Remember the to do list. Declare the value of your personal time by creating a weekend to do list—all those things you plan to do, whether it is a need or obligation or for unadulterated pleasure. There are a few important factors to consider.

First, is there time for YOU? Each weekend your first goal should be to keep a healthy balance of how you use your personal time. Being fit (in accord or harmony) is all about taking care of yourself, your responsibilities, and your needs! It can be simple. For me, a five- to ten-mile bike ride along the beach feeds my body, mind, and spirit—it is physical exercise and a relaxation of the mind. The landscape is beautiful and the air is fresh. I am reminded of and thankful for the beauty God has provided—my spirit is fed. The bike ride is pure pleasure!

Working in the garden, a round of golf with a friend, a night at the symphony, joining friends at the local pub, watching your kids play soccer, snuggling up with a good book by the fire, running with Fido, or taking the family to the zoo are just a few examples of how to get more out of life.

We all have tons of things we love to do with our free time. The problem is we don't do them! What's important is to make the commitment, choose things that do for you what bike-riding does for me—and to have a high enough regard for your personal time that you don't forsake it easily.

Next, ask yourself if your personal to do list is realistic, given the amount of time and the number of personal responsibilities you have. If not, pare it down so that it becomes something you can really commit to. When the list starts out realistically you are ahead of the game. It becomes achievable and, once achieved, you start a new pattern for your free time and are on the road to time fitness.

Negotiate your personal time when how you spend your time has an effect on the people with whom you share your life. Decide what is important and discuss your needs. After all, no one is a mind reader, and perceptions are often off base. With a clearer understanding of everyone's needs and some give and take, everyone will be better off.

Finally, don't underestimate the value of a good night's sleep. If you are sleep deprived, how can your life be in balance? Not everyone needs the same amount of sleep, but we do know when we aren't allowing enough time for a good night's sleep or if we struggle with restless nights that leave us exhausted. If your sleep habits are off kilter take a critical look at what might be wrong and what you can do about it.

If are *not* going to bed at a reasonable time for your sleep needs five out of seven nights a week, you need to put together an action plan that changes this within thirty days. Take control and recognize that everyone needs a good night's sleep.

If you repeatedly have trouble falling to sleep or your sleep is restless, seek solutions. First, when you can't sleep get up and ask yourself why. If something is on your mind, write it down on a list and face it in the morning when your mind is clear. If you always go to bed wired, think about changing your pre-bedtime activities, eliminating foods or activities that are stimulating. Replace such activities with meditation or light reading. If the cause for your sleep deprivation seems more significant, and you never wake up rested, schedule an appointment with a sleep clinic and get to the bottom of the problem.

To take proper care of yourself, it is vitally important to eat right and get a healthy dose of exercise on a regular basis. Both of these can also contribute to a better night's sleep and are essential to keeping your life in balance.

When it comes to healthy eating, apply discipline by eating the right foods at the right time. Stay away from junk food and fast-food restaurants, and eliminate snacking and late-night eating. If you must have a snack, why not have fresh fruit or vegetables?

Make exercise a habit. Too often we declare there is not enough time to dedicate to exercise—who has time to go to the gym? But there are ways to put exercise into your daily life, and twenty minutes a day or one hour three times a week is better than not exercising at all. You can achieve this with short walks in the early morning or after dinner, a ten minute morning and evening aerobic exercise routine, or getting involved in a community sports activity—the tennis team, a softball league, racquet ball, or whatever else suits you. Surely with a little thought you will discover some activity you can engage in that will add a reasonable amount of exercise to your routine and support a balanced life.

Leap of Faith

Obtaining a healthy balance takes a leap of faith and enough confidence to know that the choices you make are the right ones for you. The route to a healthy balance requires self-awareness, self-acceptance and self-care. It's a balancing act that enriches how time is spent and results in a healthier you on and off the job. ●

TAKE BACK TIME

- *Don't let work own you.*
- *Build a life of personal purpose.*
- *Feed your body, mind, and spirit.*
- *Develop healthy lifestyle boundaries.*

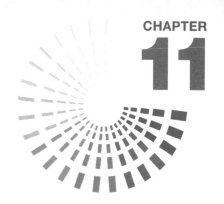

CHAPTER

11

From This Day Forward

"You never plan the future by the past."

—*Edmund Burke*

Every day we make choices. Once in a while one of those choices has an important impact on our future or on our workplace. On the other hand, many of the decisions we make each day seem insignificant; but even the seemingly insignificant decisions reflect who we are and what we value, including our time.

MAKE A DIFFERENCE

The future is yours, so go forward and don't look back. When you honor time, take care of yourself, and remove those time traps that once seemed to be the bane of your existence, life changes.

Change Habits, Change Reality

It's not easy to change the way we walk through each day and use our time. It often seems we are on automatic pilot and unable to release the control. It takes a real effort and a fair amount of discipline to change habits. But it's in our power to make changes that result in better time management.

Don't let this be just another book. Make it the impetus for you to initiate those important changes that alter your future. Start with small steps. For each of us the path is different. Some of you will want to focus on communication skills, others may need to take serious actions to become more organized, and some need to deal with poor sleep patterns. And there are those who need to stop making knee-jerk decisions that result in shouldering someone else's responsibilities, and become more effective at delegating.

Time Facts

You know the points in this book that hit home with you. Make a "My Time Facts" list of the key tips that, when employed, will have the biggest influence on changing the reality of how you manage time. Print or write the list on card stock and laminate it! Keep the list in a place where you will read it first thing in the morning. Here's an example of what a list might look like.

Of course, each person's list will be specific to their own time traps and their own life. The point is, when it is put into writing *something magical happens*. It becomes a

My Time Facts
1. Make better use of tools.
2. Take time to plan.
3. Communicate and inform.
4. Keep the monkey off my back.
5. Limit interruptions.
6. Balance my life.

commitment to change. When you look at the list each day, it reminds you that by changing habits we change our reality.

LOOK WHAT TIME CAN DO

Time is a commodity we cannot buy or save and, as previously stated, there is only so much of it. What we can do is enjoy it more by living a life of purpose. Think about what time can do for you.

More Generous Contribution

When we open up time in our busy lives we open up the opportunities to give back. We can make better use of our talents professionally and personally. We learn to be grateful, and with this comes wisdom and peace.

Professionally, you can get more involved in associations by serving in leadership positions or championing a cause. You can mentor young colleagues or subordinates to both increase their confidence and help them hone their skills.

Personally, you can be there for your family, providing direction, encouragement, and support. You can simply spend more time with family and friends, valuing all that you are to each other. You can get more involved in your church and your child's school, where volunteers are always needed.

You can provide a charitable contribution of your time to those community organizations so many people depend upon. You might run in "Race for the Cure"; play in a golf tournament that supports a cause; or volunteer with hospice, the YMCA, or another cause you feel inspired to support.

More Satisfaction

When you manage time well and your life is in balance, there is a great sense of peace about what you can accomplish and how you are living your life. You can step confidently into the future, enjoying the many aspects of your life and the people you care about. You will be, quite simply, more satisfied.

NEWFOUND FREEDOM

There is an enormous sense of freedom when we are in control of time and are content in the way we spend it. We can make time for the things we really want to do, things we may have put on the back burner for years, or perhaps something we only dreamed of doing.

Set a new course for personal or professional growth. Perhaps you always thought about going back to school to get a master's degree or start down the path of a second career. That's not such a bad idea when you consider that in the not-too-distant future people are expected to work to or beyond the age of seventy.

On the personal side, maybe you play tennis or golf but you've never taken the time to get professional assistance to master the game. You may be a swimmer or a runner, but have never taken the time to train for and enter competitions.

Why not live your dreams and pursue your passions? Maybe you've always wanted to learn how to mountain climb and reach the top of Mount Whitney. If you are creative you may have thought about becoming a musician, a writer, or a photographer. You may love cooking and fancy yourself becoming a gourmet chef. Why not begin the journey now?

Maybe it's just time to do more of what you really like to do or become even better at what you do well. It's not a novel idea, but one worth considering. It's your life, so just do it!

TAKE BACK TIME

- *Make time yours.*
- *Time is priceless—treasure it!*

"Only those that risk going too far can possibly find out how far one can go."

—*T.S. Eliot*

SUBJECT INDEX

Secrets of the Best-Run Practices Form Tool Kit BY JUDY CAPKO

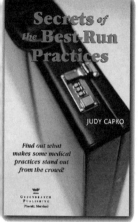

A wonderful assortment of practical time saving forms designed to help you manage your busy practice.

Each of the 44 forms below is presented in pdf. Just review, print and go!

We hope you enjoy these time-saving forms.

1. Alpha Numerical Accuracy Quiz
2. Appointment Power Words Matrix
3. Batch Control Slip
4. Charting Dos and Don'ts
5. Clinical Telephone Tracking Incoming Calls
6. Communication Matrix
7. Comparing Key Performance Indicators
8. Don't Ask These Questions
9. Employee Benefits Audit Form
10. Employee Counseling Form
11. Employee Exit Interview
12. Employment Agreement Letter
13. Guidelines For Strategic Planning
14. Individual Human Resource Record
15. Job Description Questionnaire

16. Management Skills Audit
17. Meeting Action Matrix
18. New Employee Check List
19. New Employee Progress Report
20. On Site Patient Time Study
21. Past Employer Reference Check
22. Patient Satisfaction Survey
23. Patient Visit Time Study
24. Payer Performance Table — Reimbursement per CPT Code
25. Performance Evaluation Report
26. Performance Standards Worksheet
27. Phone Tracking (Incoming calls)
28. Physician's Retreat Questionnaire
29. Pre-surgical Financial Arrangements
30. Productivity Tracking Form

31. Request For Time Off
32. Risk-Opportunity Matrix
33. Rooming Matrix — Patient Prep Standards
34. Sample Bio Sketch
35. Sample Discharge Letter
36. Sample Job Description
37. Sample Organizational Chart
38. Staff Survey — How Does Management Rate
39. Team Leader Tips
40. Telephone Appointment Tracking
41. The Art of Delegation
42. Tracking Log Diagnostic Studies
43. Training Monitor
44. Twelve Point Office Efficiency Test

With SECRETS OF THE BEST-RUN PRACTICES FORM TOOL KIT close at hand, you'll have **everything you need to know** to run an efficient and successful practice.

GREENBRANCH PUBLISHING

ORDER TODAY! Only $29.95! *(plus $4.95 shipping & handling)*

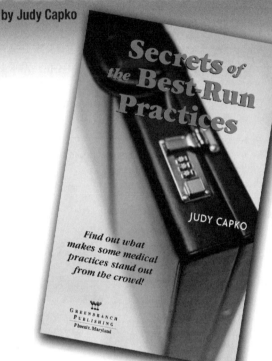
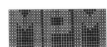